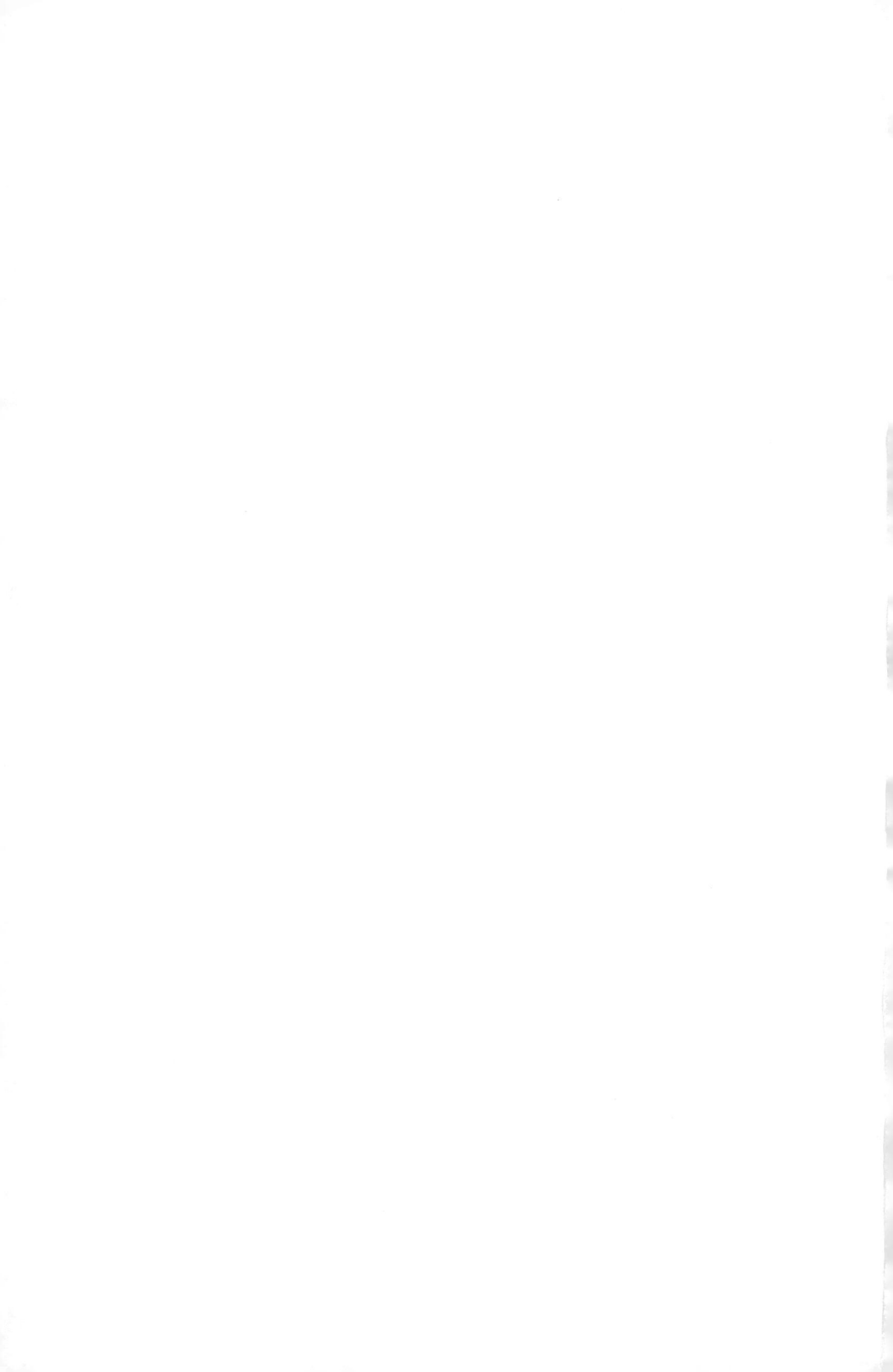

Springer Series on Geriatric Nursing

Mathy D. Mezey, RN, EdD, FAAN, Series Editor

Advisory Board: Margaret Dimond, PhD, RN, FAAN; Steven H. Ferris, PhD; Terry Fulmer, RN, PhD, FAAN; Linda Kaeser, PhD, RN, ACSW, FAAN; Virgene Kayser-Jones, PhD, RN, FAAN; Eugenia Siegler, MD; Neville E. Strumpf, PhD, RN, FAAN; May Wykle, PhD, RN, FAAN; Mary K. Walker, PhD, RN, FAAN

2002	**Prostate Cancer: Nursing Assessment, Management, and Care** *Meredith Wallace, PhD, RN, CS-ANP, and Lorrie L Powel, PhD, RN*
2002	**Bathing Without a Battle: Personal Care of Individuals With Dementia** *Ann Louise Barrick, PhD, Joanne Rader, RN, MN, FAAN, Beverly Hoeffer, DNSc, RN, FAAN, and Philip D. Sloane, MD, MPH*
2001	**Critical Care Nursing of the Elderly, Second Edition** *Terry T. Fulmer, PhD, RN, FAAN, Marquis D. Foreman, PhD, RN, FAAN, and Mary Walker, PhD, RN, FAAN, and Kristen S. Montgomery, PhD, RNC, IBCLC*
1999	**Geriatric Nursing Protocols for Best Practice** *Ivo Abraham, PhD, RN, FAAN, Melissa M. Bottrell, MPH, Terry T. Fulmer, PhD, RN, FAAN, and Mathy D. Mezey, EdD, RN, FAAN*
1998	**Home Care for Older Adults: A guide for Families and Other Caregivers—Text and Instructor's Manual** *Mary Ann Rosswurm, EdD, RN, CS, FAAN*
1998	**Restraint-Free Care: Individualized Approaches for Frail Elders** *Neville E. Strumpf, PhD, RN, C, FAAN, Joanne Patterson Robinson, PhD, RN, Joan Stockman Wagner, MSN, CRNP, and Lois K. Evans, DNSc, RN, FAAN*
1996	**Gerontology Review Guide for Nurses** *Elizabeth Chapman Shaid, RN, MSN, CRNP, and Kay Huber, DEd, RN, CRNP*
1995	**Strengthening Geriatric Nursing Education** *Terry T. Fulmer, RN, PhD, FAAN, and Marianne Marzo, PhD, RN, CS*
1994	**Nurse-Physician Collaboration: Care of Adults and the Elderly** *Eugenia L. Siegler, MD, and Fay W. Whitney, PhD, RN, FAAN*
1993	**Health Assessment of the Older Individual, Second Edition** *Mathy Doval Mezey, RN, EdD, FAAN, Shirlee Ann Stokes, RN, EdD, FAAN, and Louise Hartnett Rauckhorst, RNC, ANP, EdD*
1992	**Critical Care Nursing of the Elderly** *Terry T. Fulmer, RN, PhD, FAAN, and Mary K. Walker, PhD, RN, FAAN*

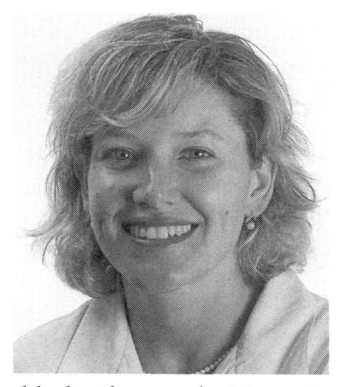

Meredith Wallace, PhD, RN, CS-ANP, has been a nurse since she completed her BSN degree at Boston University, Magna Cum Laude in 1988. Following this, she earned an MSN in medical-surgical nursing with a specialty in geriatrics from Yale University and a PhD in nursing research and theory development at New York University. She is currently an Assistant Professor at Southern Connecticut State University, Department of Nursing. She has lectured widely throughout the United States on issues pertinent to the care of the elderly. She was the Managing Editor of the *Journal Applied Nursing Research,* and is the author of several journal articles and book chapters. She most recently worked as Associate Editor of the *The Geriatric Nursing Research Digest,* which won the *American Journal of Nursing* Book of the Year Award. Her research focuses on the quality of life of older men receiving watchful waiting for prostate cancer. She lives in New Haven, Connecticut with her husband and two children.

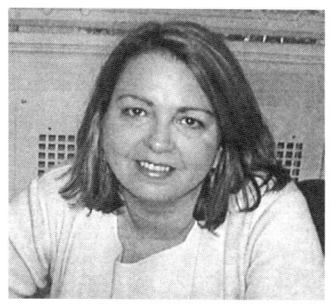

Lorrie L. Powel, PhD, RN, is currently a postdoctoral fellow at the Boston University School of Public Health and the Center for Health Quality, Outcomes, and Economic Research at the Edith Nourse Rogers Memorial Veterans Hospital, Bedford, Massachusetts. She recently completed her doctoral degree at the University of Maryland School of Nursing, where she received a dissertation award from the Health Care Financing Administration for her research focusing on the impact of postprostectomy urinary incontinence on psychosocial adjustment to illness and quality of life. Her current research, funded by the Department of Defense, will continue to explore postprostatectomy incontinence with a focus on ethnic identity. During the past several decades Dr. Powel has been a frequent contributor to the oncology nursing literature focusing on issues of quality of life and the management of treatment-related symptoms in patients with cancer.

Prostate Cancer

Nursing Assessment, Management, and Care

Meredith Wallace, PhD, RN, CS-ANP
Lorrie L. Powel, PhD, RN, Editors

Springer Publishing Company

Copyright © 2002 by Springer Publishing Company, Inc.

All rights reserved

No part of this publication may be reproduced, stored in a retrieval system, or transmitted in any form or by any means, electronic, mechanical, photocopying, recording, or otherwise, without the prior permission of Springer Publishing Company, Inc.

Springer Publishing Company, Inc.
536 Broadway
New York, NY 10012-3955

Acquisitions Editor: Sheri W. Sussman
Production Editor: Jean Hurkin-Torres
Cover design by Susan Hauley

02 03 04 05 06 / 5 4 3 2 1

Library of Congress Cataloging-in-Publication Data

Prostate cancer : nursing assessment, management, and care / Meredith Wallace, Lorri L. Powel, editors.
    p. ; cm. — (Springer series on geriatric nursing)
    Includes bibliographical references and index.
    ISBN 0-8261-8745-5
    1. Prostate—Cancer—Nursing. I. Wallace, Meredith, PhD, RN, II. Powel, Lorrie L., PhD, RN. III. Series
    [DNLM: 1. Prostatic Neoplasms—nursing. 2. Nursing Assessment. WJ 752 P96553 47 2002]
    RC280.P7 P7594 2002
    616.99'463—dc21

                                                  2001057650

Printed in the United States of America by Maple-Vail.

CONTENTS

Contributors		*vii*
Foreword		*ix*
1	Prostate Cancer: The Nature of the Problem *Meredith Wallace and Lorrie L. Powel*	1
2	Prostate Cancer: Risk Factors and Prevention *Joannie Meehan*	14
3	Assessment, Screening and Diagnosis of Prostate Cancer *Eun-Hyun Lee*	33
4	Treatment Choices and the Decision-Making Process *Maureen E. O'Rourke*	46
5	Quality of Life with Prostate Cancer *Lorrie L. Powel and Meredith Wallace*	62
6	Nursing Care for Radical Prostatectomy *Penny Marschke*	77
7	Nursing Care for Radiation Treatment *Vanna M. Dest*	89
8	Hormone Therapy *Dorothy A. Calabrese*	110
9	Watchful Waiting—Managing Prostate Cancer as a Chronic Disease *Meredith Wallace*	126

10	Prevalent Issues in Patient Education *Vanna M. Dest and Meredith Wallace*	140
11	End of Life Care *Susan Derby and Diane B. Loseth*	153

References   *173*

Index   *215*

CONTRIBUTORS

Dorothy A. Calabrese, MSN, RN, CURN, CNP
Nurse Practitioner/Clinical Nurse Specialist—Urology Oncology
Taussig Cancer Center
Cleveland Clinic Foundation
Cleveland, OH

Susan Derby, RN, MA, CGNP
Pain and Palliative Care Service
Department of Neurology
Memorial Sloan-Kettering Cancer Center
New York, NY

Vanna M. Dest, MSN, APRN, CS, AOCN
Radiation Oncology Clinical Nurse Specialist
Hospital of Saint Raphael
New Haven, CT

Eun-Hyun Lee, RN, PhD
Division of Nursing Science
Ajou University
South Korea

Diane B. Loseth, RN, MSN, OCN
Pain and Palliative Care Service
Department of Neurology
Memorial Sloan-Kettering Cancer Center
New York, NY

Penny Marschke, RN, PhD
Clinical Research Program Manager
Brady Urological Institute
Johns Hopkins University
Baltimore, MD

Joannie Meehan, APRN, CS, MSN, AOCN
Oncology Nurse Practitioner
Medical Oncology
University of Connecticut Health Center
Farmington, CT

Maureen O'Rourke, RN, PhD
Assistant Professor, School of Nursing
University of North Carolina
Greensboro, NC

and

Adjunct Assistant Professor of Medicine—Hematology/Oncology
Wake Forest University School of Medicine
Winston-Salem, NC

FOREWORD

Prostate cancer is the most commonly diagnosed malignancy and the second leading cause of cancer death in men (Haas & Sakr, 1997). Prostate cancer, however, does not follow a predictable clinical path. Less than one third of men diagnosed with prostate cancer will ultimately die from this disease (Holmboe & Concato, 2000).

Incidence, that is, new cases, of prostate cancer differ between Caucasian men and non-Caucasian men, 107.3 per 100,000 and 145.8 per 100,000, respectively (Kassabian & Graham, 1995). The reason for the difference is not clear and warrants further investigation. Factors associated with incident cases include increased public awareness and detection, environmental factors such as exposure to cadmium, genetic factors, and high fat diets (Kassabian & Graham, 1995). It has been estimated that half of the men who survive to 85 years of age have evidence of prostate cancer (Agency for Health Care Policy and Research, 1995). As the baby boom generation continues to age, the absolute number of men with diagnosed prostate cancer will increase. Radical prostatectomy remains the gold standard treatment, although other options are available to men and their physicians. It may be a result of earlier detection and effective treatment that death rates from prostate cancer have been declining over the last several years. Thus, more men will survive the diagnosis and treatment of prostate cancer than ever before.

There is a human face behind the facts and figures. In his elegantly moving memoir about prostate cancer, *Man to Man*, Michael Korda (1996) says, "Just as breast cancer is the biggest fear of most women—formerly unspoken, but no longer—prostate cancer is the biggest fear of most men. It carries with it not only the fear of dying, like all cancer, but fears that go to the very core of masculinity . . ." (p. 3). Prostate cancer treatment may mean ultimate cure for men, but it may also bring devastating and lasting after-effects of incontinence and impotence. Men and their partners, therefore, face difficult decisions after diagnosis. Holmboe and Concato (2000) reported the results of a study investigating men's treatment decisions. They found that men relied on their own weighing of evidence rather than recommendations of their physician. Men often rejected watchful waiting because of their need to "do something" to remove the cancer; family members needs were also taken into consideration when watchful waiting was rejected. Men do weigh the track record of treatments, the risk of complications, their impressions of invasiveness or duration of treatments, and likelihood of having future treatment options.

The information contained in this text is of vital importance as more men face screening, assessment, diagnosis, and treatment of prostate cancer. Nurses who assess and provide care for these men need to be fully informed about the epidemiology and pathophysiology of prostate cancer. The latest evidence about options will help men make treatment decisions. Understanding the impact of prostate cancer and its treatment on the quality of life cannot be underestimated in its importance. Most men will survive prostate cancer. Some, however, will die from this disease despite the best efforts of physicians and nurses caring for them. As nurses, we need to understand the physical and psychological needs of both groups and do our best to meet them. Prostate cancer should no longer remain the unspoken fear among men.

MARY H. PALMER, PHD, RNC, FAAN
Associate Professor and Director, Office of Research
Rutgers, The State University of New Jersey
College of Nursing

REFERENCES

Agency for Health Care Policy and Research (1995). Patient outcomes research team. Prostate Cancer. AHCPR Pub No. 95-N010. U.S. Department of Health and Human Services. Public Health Service.

Haas, G., & Sakr, W. (1997). Epidemiology of prostate cancer. *CA—A Cancer Journal for Clinicians, 47*(5), 273–287.

Holmboe, E., & Concato, J. (2000). Treatment decisions for localized prostate cancer. *Journal of General Internal Medicine, 15*(10), 694–701.

Kassabian, V., & Graham, S. (1995). Urologic and male genital cancers. In G. Murphy, W. Lawrence, & R. Lenhard (Eds.), *American Cancer Society textbook on clinical oncology.* Atlanta, GA: The American Cancer Society.

Korda, M. (1996). *Man to man: Surviving prostate cancer.* New York: Random House.

1
Prostate Cancer: The Nature of the Problem

Meredith Wallace and Lorrie L. Powel

Prostate cancer is defined as a malignant tumor within the prostate gland (Garnick, 1994). It is the most common form of cancer in American adult males in all age groups and currently surpasses the incidence of lung cancer in this country. It is the second leading cause of death from cancer in men in the United States (U.S.). Current estimates are that 8% of all men in the U.S. will be diagnosed with prostate cancer during their lifetime. The cause of prostate cancer is not known. Environmental factors such as exposure to cadmium and zinc (Haas & Sakr, 1997), Western diet, and infectious agents transmitted through sexual activity have also been linked to prostate cancer. However, other factors such as age, race, familial factors, and genetic predisposition are also hypothesized to play a role.

This chapter will provide the background for the problem of prostate cancer in the U.S. and its significance for nurses. The epidemiology of prostate cancer, its pervasive nature in today's society and the pathophysiology of the disease will be presented. In addition, the information presented herein will be used as a framework within which the content of the book is introduced.

EPIDEMIOLOGY

Exploring the epidemiology of prostate cancer is a useful way to develop an understanding of the description and impact of the disease on the population. Much of the information contained within this chapter is based on data collected and reported by the Surveillance, Epidemiology, and End Results (SEER) program. The SEER program was created in 1973 by the National Cancer Institute (NCI) to provide an estimate of cancer incidence and prevalence in the U.S. It consists of nine national data collection sites, representing approximately 14% of the U.S. population (SEER, 2000).

Incidence

Overall, the sixth most common cancer in the world, prostate cancer is ranked as the fourth most common cancer among males worldwide (Parkin, Pisani, & Ferlay, 1999). In the U.S. it is the most prevalent cancer in men, with 198,000 new cases estimated in 2001 (Greenlee, Hill-Harmon, Murray, & Thun, 2001). Interestingly, North America has the highest incidence in the world, in contrast to China where men are at little risk (92.39 vs. 1.08 per 100,000, respectively) (Parkin et al., 1999).

Prostate cancer is a malignancy that was once detected only in late stages, resulting in imminent death (Litwin, 1994). More recently, intensive screening efforts, use of prostate specific antigen (PSA), and the diagnosis of asymptomatic, latent cancers in the U.S. and other developed countries have resulted in both increased reports of the disease (incidence) and increased numbers of men living with the disease (prevalence) (Newschaffer, 1997). In fact, the incidence of prostate cancer in the U.S. doubled in the 10-year period from 1984 to 1994 (Parkin et al., 1999), largely due to intensive screening efforts with PSA. Figure 1.1 shows that the dramatic increase in prostate cancer incidence over the last several decades. As the life expectancy of the male population increases over time, the incidence and prevalence of prostate cancer is expected to further increase.

Prevalence

The slow-growing nature of prostate tumors accounts for the high prevalence of prostate cancer and its proclivity for survival. The five-year relative survival rate for prostate cancer has increased from 45.1% for men diagnosed in 1973 to 66.9% for men diagnosed in 1990. The relative survival rate depends largely on the stage of disease at diagnosis; most men are diagnosed early with localized prostate cancer (SEER, 2000).

The increased survival rate has resulted in greater numbers of men living with prostate cancer. Both the increased incidence and prevalence of the disease underscore the need for knowledgeable and competent nurses to care for these men as they go through diagnosis, make treatment decisions,

The Nature of the Problem 3

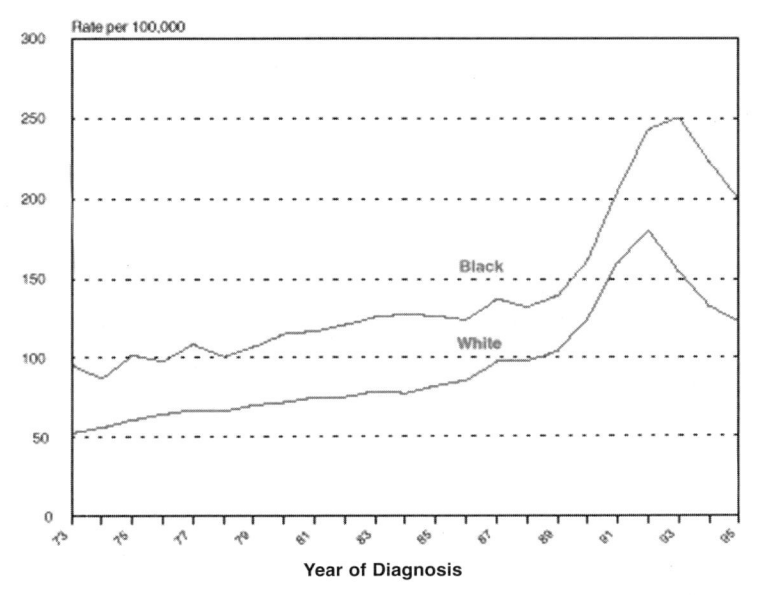

Rates are age adjusted to the 1970 U.S. standard. Rates from 1973–1987 are based on data from the 9 standard SEER registries. Data from San Jose and Los Angeles are included in the rate calculations for 1988–1995.

FIGURE 1.1 Prostate cancer SEER incidence rates, 1973–1995.

and manage both the symptoms of the disease and side effects of treatment. This book premieres as a resource in providing information on the nursing assessment, diagnosis, treatment, and care of men with prostate cancer.

AFFECTED POPULATIONS

More than any other cancer, prostate cancer is known for its characteristic rise in incidence with age. It is estimated that half of the men who survive to 85 years of age have evidence of prostate cancer (AHCPR, 1995). While the disease does strike men in their fourth and fifth decades, over 81% of cases occur in men over age 65 worldwide (Parkin et al., 1999); the median age is 66 years (Scher, Isaacs, Fuks, & Walsh, 1995). The age distribution is displayed in Figure 1.2. The advanced age of men with prostate cancer precipitates the need for nurses to be knowledgeable regarding oncology and geriatric nursing assessment and management practices.

Age at Diagnosis

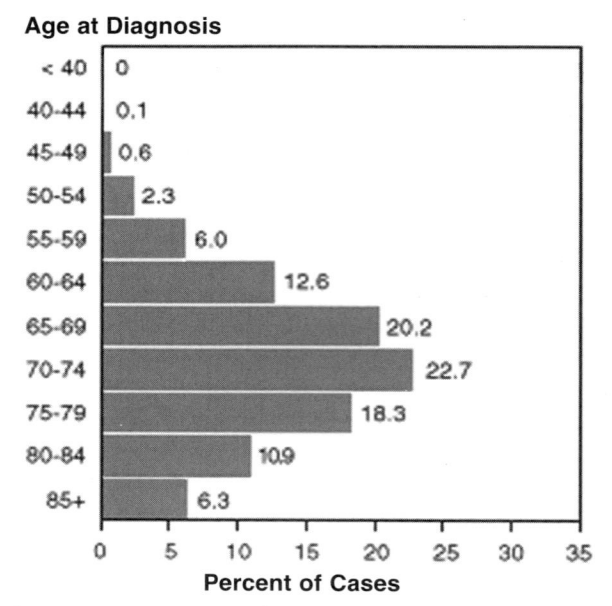

Age	Percent
< 40	0
40-44	0.1
45-49	0.6
50-54	2.3
55-59	6.0
60-64	12.6
65-69	20.2
70-74	22.7
75-79	18.3
80-84	10.9
85+	6.3

Percent of Cases

* Data from San Jose-Monterey and Los Angeles used only for 1988–1995.

FIGURE 1.2   Prostate cancer cases: Distribution by age, SEER Program*, 1973–1995.

The geographic range in the incidence of prostate cancer varies widely with higher incidence rates in the U.S. than in all other countries. The smallest incidence occurs in China (SEER, 2000). While the high incidence in the U.S. may be partially explained by the widespread use of prostate cancer screening throughout the country, studies of men migrating to the U.S. from countries with a lower incidence show an increase in prostate cancer as they become acclimated to the U.S. This suggests other risk factors uniquely present in the U.S.—for example, high fat content in the Western diet. In a study of 51,529 U.S. men, Giovanucci and colleagues (1993) found that total fat consumption was directly related to risk of advanced prostate cancer. Risk factors for development of prostate cancer will be more fully discussed in chapter 2. Figure 1.3 details the incidence of prostate cancer worldwide. The global occurrence of prostate cancer, and the potential impact of migrating to the U.S. with the disease, underscores the need for culturally competent nursing care for men with prostate cancer.

The incidence of prostate cancer varies by race, with the highest number of cases seen among White men. Table 1.1 shows the incidence of

The Nature of the Problem 5

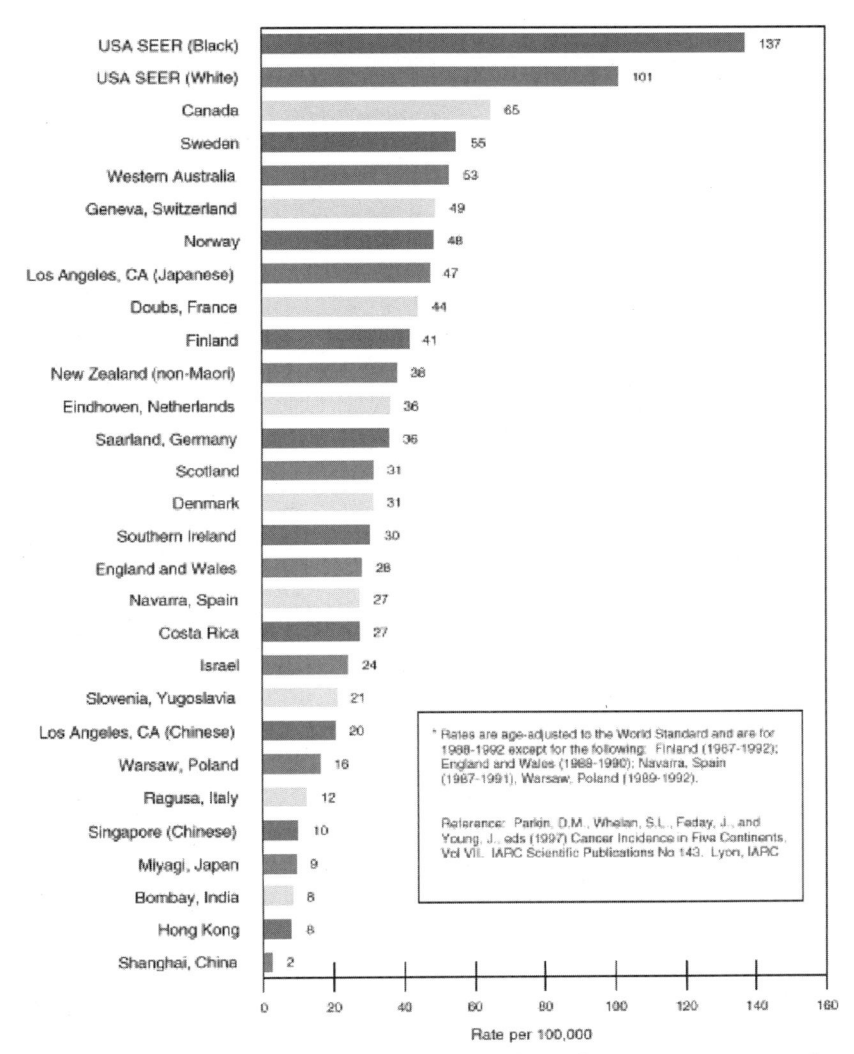

FIGURE 1.3 Prostate cancer international incidence rates*. Reproduced with permission (SEER, 2000).

prostate cancer by race. SEER data (2000) indicate that the mortality rate among Whites is 34%, compared to 123% for Blacks. Incidence rates are highest for Blacks and lowest for Native Americans. The disparity in incidence and mortality rates among Blacks is of great concern because of its enormous implications. Indeed, the reduction of ethnic disparity in prostate cancer has been identified as a priority goal of Healthy People 2010 (www.health.gov/healthypeople).

TABLE 1.1 Prostate Cancer Cases: Distribution by Race, SEER Program*, 1973–1995

Race	Number	Percent
White	228,602	83.8
Black	28,172	10.3
Asians	9,721	3.6
Japanese	3,489	1.3
Filipino	3,014	1.1
Chinese	1,880	0.7
Hawaiian	594	0.2
Korean	158	0.1
Other Asian	586	0.2
Native American	466	0.2
Other race	390	0.1
Unknown	5,338	2.0
Total	272,689	100.0

* Data from San Jose-Monterey and Los Angeles used only for 1988–1995.

PATHOPHYSIOLOGY OF PROSTATE CANCER

Anatomy and Physiology

In the adult male, the prostate gland is a walnut-shaped structure (4–6 cm long) made up of glandular and muscular material enclosed within a fibrous capsule. Its primary role is to produce part of the fluid for semen ejaculated during orgasm. Located at the base of the bladder neck, it encircles the urethra, a small portion of which passes through the prostate. This is referred to as the prostatic urethra. The prostate is posterior to the symphysis pubis and to the fore of the rectum. Adjacent to the prostate are the seminal vesicles, two small sacs where semen is stored.

The prostate is made up of distinct zones including the peripheral, central, and transition zones. These designations are based on their morphology, ductal pattern, and embryonic origin (Morse & Resnick, 1990). Typically, two conditions may come about as a result of the enlargement of the prostate in aging men—benign prostatic hyperplasia (BPH), which occurs in the central or transitional zone, and prostate cancer, which most often originates in the peripheral zone. However, the mechanisms that dictate prostate growth and differentiation are poorly understood. Both benign growth (as in BPH) and prostate cancer are androgen dependent and originate locally within the prostate. Little is known about the actual inter- and intra-cellular communication that directs androgen-receptor mediated gene activities during different phases of cell proliferation.

Adding to our lack of understanding of carcinogenesis, the mechanisms of cancer cell invasion, migration, and metastasis are also poorly understood. The heterogeneous growth pattern of prostate cancer creates an appearance of three different diseases: 1) a rapidly growing virulent disease; 2) a latent subclinical innocuous disease; and 3) a slow but clinically progressive disease (von Eschenbach, 1999).

These properties, along with the lack of insight into the biological and molecular behavior of this disease, have contributed to difficulty in developing specific screening mechanisms and identifying successful treatment—in short, reducing mortality. It is known that adenocarcinoma—the most common histological type of prostate cancer—typically metastasizes locally via the blood vessels and lymphatics to the seminal vesicles, lymph nodes, bladder, and peritoneum (Lind, Kravitz, & Greig, 1993). Lymphatic extension can continue through the pelvis and travel to the thoracic and supraclavicular regions. Hematogenous spread characteristically includes the lungs, liver, kidney, and bones (Lind et al., 1993).

STAGING

Classification systems are used to characterize the degree of aggressiveness of the tumor (i.e., invasion of tissue, node involvement, and metastases to other tissue). Two anatomic staging systems are commonly used to classify prostate cancers in the United States. The Jewett system (stages A–D), now referred to as the Whitmore-Jewett staging system, was first described in 1975 (Jewett, 1975). In 1997, the American Joint Committee on Cancer (AJCC) and the International Union Against Cancer (UICC) developed a revised TNM (tumor, node, metastasis) classification system which expanded on the TNM system originally devised in the late 1980s to include subcategories of the T stage (AJCC, 1997). Both the Jewett and TNM systems will be presented here.

Within the Jewett system, stage A is clinically undetectable and characterized as three or fewer well differentiated foci (A1), or greater than three, or diffuse foci and poorly differentiated (A2). Stage B tumors are clinically palpable. They are characterized as < 1.5 cm involving one lobe only (B2) or > 1.5 cm and diffusely involved (B2). Stage C designates extension beyond the prostatic capsule, but without local or distant metastasis. Stage D is consistent with evidence of metastatic disease. It is divided into two substages: D1 includes extension into the pelvic nodes below the aortic bifurcation; D2 designates lymph node involvement above the aortic bifurcation and/or distant metastasis. The TNM classification is delineated in Table 1.2.

TABLE 1.2 TNM Staging Definitions

Primary tumor (T)

TX: Primary tumor cannot be assessed
T0: No evidence of primary tumor
T1: Clinically inapparent tumor not palpable nor visible by imaging
T1a: Tumor incidental histologic finding in 5% or less of tissue resected
T1b: Tumor incidental histologic finding in more than 5% of tissue resected
T1c: Tumor identified by needle biopsy (e.g., because of elevated PSA)
T2: Tumor confined within prostate*
T2a: Tumor involves one lobe
T2b: Tumor involves both lobes
T3: Tumor extends through the prostatic capsule**
T3a: Extracapsular extension (unilateral or bilateral)
T3b: Tumor invades seminal vesicle(s)
T4: Tumor is fixed or invades adjacent structures other than seminal vesicles: bladder neck, external sphincter, rectum, levator muscles, and/or pelvic wall

Regional lymph nodes (N)

Regional lymph nodes are the nodes of the true pelvis, which essentially are the pelvic nodes below the bifurcation of the common iliac arteries. Distant lymph nodes are outside the confines of the true pelvis and their involvement constitutes distant metastasis.

NX: Regional lymph nodes cannot be assessed
N0: No regional lymph node metastasis
N1: Metastasis in regional lymph node or nodes

*Distant metastasis*** (M)*

MX: Distant metastasis cannot be assessed
M0: No distant metastasis
M1: Distant metastasis
M1a: Nonregional lymph node(s)
M1b: Bone(s)
M1c: Other site(s)

* Tumor found in one or both lobes by needle biopsy, but not palpable or reliably visible by imaging, is classified as T1c.
** Invasion into the prostatic apex or into (but not beyond) the prostatic capsule is not classified as T3, but as T2.
*** When more than one site of metastasis is present, the most advanced category (pM1c) is used.
Note: From American Joint Commission on Cancer (1998). *Cancer Staging Manual 5th Edition.* Chicago, IL: Author.

CELLULAR CLASSIFICATION

The overwhelming majority (95%) of all prostate cancers are adenocarcinomas. Sarcoma, ductal, and transitional cell carcinomas occur rarely (Frank, Graham, & Nabors, 1991). In addition to the anatomic classification systems previously identified, a histopathologic system is also used to classify tumors. The Gleason grading system is based on the tumor's glandular differentiation and growth pattern. Degree of tumor differentiation and abnormality of histologic growth pattern are typically associated with likelihood of metastases and with death (Albertsen, Hanley, Gleason, & Barry, 1998). That is, if a cancer looks similar to a normal cell, it is well differentiated, and therefore likely to be less aggressive. A poorly differentiated cancer (looks like an immature cell) is likely to be more aggressive. Gleason scores range from one to five, with one being the most differentiated and five being the least differentiated. The actual Gleason score is based on the sum of two scores of the two most poorly differentiated parts of the tumor, and can therefore range from 2 to 10, with the higher score associated with a poorer prognosis.

Gleason scores, coupled with PSA and age, have been found to be strong predictors of metastatic disease. Researchers have learned that men 70 years of age and older with a PSA greater than 20 ng/ml and a Gleason score of 8 to 10 had an 85% chance of having metastatic disease. Men 50 years and younger with PSAs less than 4 ng/ml and a Gleason score of less than 7 had a 24% chance of having extracapsular disease (Gilliland et al., 1999).

Risk Factors

There is a greater incidence of prostate cancer in the male relatives of men who died from the disease. Hereditary prostate cancer is autosomal dominant characterized by early disease onset. Because autosomal dominant inheritance of the disease is well-accepted, there is currently strong support for the screening of first-degree relatives of men with prostate cancer, particularly male relatives who developed the disease at an early age and those with a strong positive family history of the disease. There is no doubt that the earlier prostate cancer is diagnosed, the more favorable the prognosis will be. Family history, as well as other modifiable and non-modifiable risk factors will be discussed in chapter 2. Nursing interventions for reducing modifiable risk factors will also be presented.

Screening, Assessment, and Diagnosis

Early and effective assessment of the disease, especially in the U.S., impacts the mortality of prostate cancer. The PSA is the best serum marker for prostate cancer available today, however, its use in mass screening is hotly debated. The PSA detects both benign and malignant prostate disease. In fact, studies have demonstrated that many patients with BPH have had abnormal PSA levels; however, because of its application in the management of prostate cancer, a PSA level is commonly drawn when prostate cancer is suspected. An elevated PSA level, that is > 10 ng/mL, indicates a 66% probability of cancer (Kassabian & Graham, 1995). PSA not only detects clinically identifiable cancers, but it has also been instrumental in identifying subclinical tumors.

Men with prostate cancer may be asymptomatic at first, but early symptoms tend to be those of lower urinary tract obstruction—hesitancy, post-void dribbling, decreased force of stream, and feeling of incomplete bladder emptying. These may also be symptoms of BPH. Hematuria is rare. Symptoms of bladder outlet obstruction, ureteral obstruction with possible anuria, azotemia, uremia, anemia, and anorexia are indicative of advanced presentation (Frank et al., 1991). Bone pain is the most frequent complaint of men who present with metastatic disease.

A history and physical exam is important in identifying symptoms of prostate cancer. The digital rectal examination remains the gold standard for detection, however, diagnosis is made by histologic or cytologic confirmation. This is commonly accomplished through needle biopsy or fine needle aspiration of suspicious nodules or an indurated area of the prostate. Biopsies are often guided by transurethral ultrasound (TRUS), which uses sound waves from a small rectal probe to translate images of the prostate to a computer screen. In-depth discussion of the controversy and merits of PSA as well as other assessment techniques and diagnostic tests will be extensively discussed in chapter 3.

Quality of Life

Quality of life (QOL) of men has gained increased attention as a significant factor in the management of cancer and cancer-related problems. The personal nature of QOL and the great variability inherent in individual values make defining the concept difficult. Decision making regarding prostate cancer treatment as well as living with the disease, managing the symptoms and side effects of treatment all impact the QOL of men with prostate cancer. The impact of prostate cancer on QOL will be discussed extensively in chapter five.

Treatment Decision-Making and Approaches

Several treatment approaches available to men with prostate cancer are discussed in this book. The vast array of treatment choices often places physicians and patients into highly critical analysis before choosing the best treatment. The decision-making process and the factors identified in making that process are covered in chapter four. Radical prostatectomy and radiation therapy are the two most common treatment methods for patients with tumors confined to the prostate gland. These approaches to treating prostate cancer will be discussed extensively in chapters 7 and 8, respectively. These treatments are recommended for patients with life expectancies greater than 10 years. Watchful waiting is the treatment strategy for men over the age of 70 with low-grade tumors, no symptoms, and other chronic illnesses. Watchful waiting as a treatment option, and the nursing care associated with it, will be presented in chapter 9. Androgen ablation therapy is the treatment of choice for the care of patients whose prostate cancer has spread beyond the prostate gland. This and other methods of hormonal therapy will be discussed in chapter eight. Figure 1.4 shows the percentage of men in the U.S. receiving each treatment option.

Mortality

Despite the increased incidence of prostate cancer, deaths from possible cancer declined from 34,902 in 1994 to 32,891 in 1997 (Greenlee, Murray,

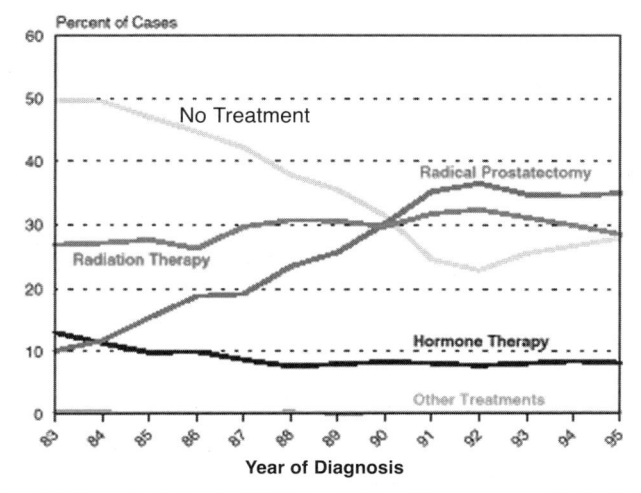

Note: Based on data from the 9 standard SEER registries. Rates are age-adjusted to the 1970 U.S. standard.

FIGURE 1.4 Prostate cancer SEER distribution of cases by treatment (1983–1995).

Bilden, & Wingo, 2000). This stability in death rate is due partly to both the earlier detection of the disease as well as advances in prostate cancer treatment. Figure 1.5 shows the mortality rates in the United States from 1990 through 1995. Fair, Fleshner, and Heston (1997) reported that the average risk of dying from prostate cancer is 3.5% for White men and 4.46% for Black men. Overall, it is estimated that 31,900 men died of prostate cancer in the year 2000 (Greenlee, Hill-Harmon, Murray, & Thun, 2001).

Despite the stable mortality rate of prostate cancer, nurses often care for men in their final stages of the disease. End-of-life care for men with

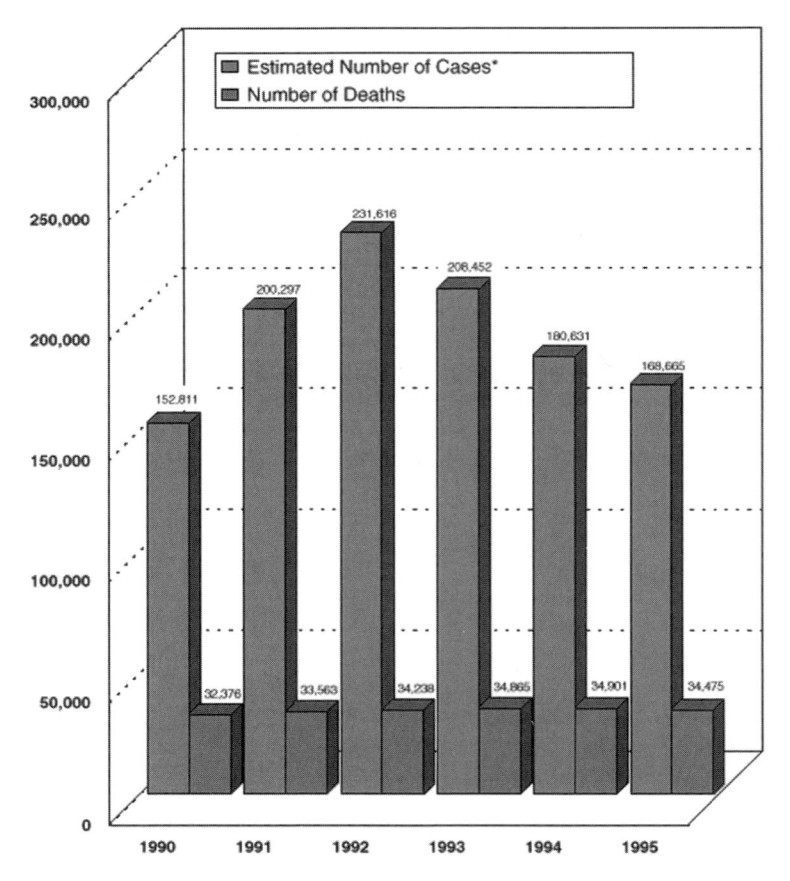

* Estimates obtained by multiplying the age-specific incidence rates for the 11 SEER registries by the U.S. population for each year.

FIGURE 1.5 SEER prostate cancer incidence and mortality rates in the U.S. from 1990 to 1995.

prostate cancer involves the management of the complex symptoms of the disease, including fatigue, anemia, lymphedema, hydronephrosis, anxiety, and depression. The care of the man dying of prostate cancer will be presented in chapter 10.

SUMMARY

The increased incidence and prevalence of prostate cancer have resulted in a larger number of men requiring nursing care for the disease. Prostate cancer presents many clinical challenges to the nurse. Understanding risk factors, appropriate use of screening and assessment techniques, treatment decision-making, and managing the complex symptoms and side effects of treatment are among those clinical challenges. The contents of this book, developed by clinical nurse experts, provides previously undocumented information on state-of-the art care of men with prostate cancer. Competent nursing care will assist the large numbers of men diagnosed and living with the disease each day to live the highest possible quality of life.

2

Prostate Cancer: Risk Factors and Prevention

Joannie Meehan

The Oncology Nursing Society (ONS)/American Nurses' Association (ANA) Standards of Oncology Nursing Practice identify 11 high-incidence problem areas common to patients with cancer (1996). The purpose of these standards is to serve as a guide to providing uniform, quality care and to serve as a basis to facilitate and evaluate professional nursing development (Volker, 1998). Prevention and early detection are the focus of the first standard of care addressed by the ONS/ANA. Although separate entities, prevention and early detection both serve to reduce the morbidity and mortality of cancer. The ONS recently published a supplement to the *Oncology Nursing Forum* (Carroll-Johnson, Mahon, & Jennings-Dozier, 2000) devoted to considerations facing oncology nurses involved in cancer prevention and detection.

Disease prevention utilizing risk reduction strategies continues to gain attention in the medical literature and the news media. The disappointing attempts at disease eradication and control through administration of anti-tumor therapies (i.e., chemotherapy, radiation therapy, surgery, etc.) encourage this approach. The National Cancer Institute (NCI) has made prevention research a high priority. In 1999 alone the NCI evaluated over 400 chemoprevention agents; more than 40 of these are now in ongoing clinical trials.

Prevention strategies include primary, secondary, and tertiary approaches. Primary prevention involves reducing or eliminating the risk of disease in individuals or groups who do not yet exhibit symptoms of disease. Primary prevention decreases the likelihood that a healthy individual or population will contract an illness through use of health promotion strategies and prevention recommendations. Secondary prevention involves reducing or eliminating the risk of disease in those considered at high risk for the disease, including those with precursor lesions (e.g., cervical dysplasia, carcinoma-in-situ of the breast, colonic polyps). It consists of early diagnosis, early detection, screening, and treatment of early stages of disease. Tertiary prevention minimizes morbidity by preventing complications that result from permanent or irreversible disease (Loescher, 1997).

A risk factor is an element of personal behavior, genetic makeup, or exposure that is statistically associated with an increased frequency of a person's chance of developing a disease. It is important to remember that although risk factors may increase a person's chance of developing a disease, they do not always result in disease; conversely, others who have the disease may have no known risk factors. The nurse must have a thorough understanding of risk factors before she/he can provide information or make recommendations for risk reduction. Risk assessment is a procedure by which the probability of a person's development of disease, disability, or death is predicted through analysis of individual risk factors (Olsen, Morrison, & Ashley, 1998).

Nurses are in a unique position to assess the combinations of risk factors which identify subpopulations of clients at high risk (e.g., lifestyle factors, occupational and environmental risks, biologic risk factors, iatrogenic risks, and other contributing factors). Once identified, measures for risk reduction and early detection can be employed. Informed and knowledgeable nurses can provide information about risk factors and risk reduction measures in their role as educator. They can also provide direction and moral support for adherence to lifestyle changes and participate in research through identification of clients for entry onto research protocols and through pertinent data collection.

A man's risk of developing prostate cancer is influenced by both genetic and environmental factors. Most of the known risk factors are constitutional and cannot be controlled (e.g., age, race, and family history of prostate cancer). The contribution of modifiable factors (e.g., lifestyle or environment) to the incidence of prostate cancer has been studied and supported by recent investigations (Giovannucci, 1996). The fact that subclinical (i.e., asymptomatic) rates are fairly consistent worldwide, while clinically significant (i.e., symptomatic) rates vary, supports the hypothesis that environmental and lifestyle factors may contribute to the promotion of prostate cancer (Doherty & Breslin, 1996). Based on what is currently known or suspected to cause cancer in the United States, it is estimated that environmental factors may contribute to up to 80% of all cancers (Johnson, 1998).

HISTORICAL PERSPECTIVE, CONTEMPORARY FOCUS, AND REVIEW OF ISSUES

Many proposed risk reduction measures for cancer prevention and control have been identified over the past several decades through improved methods in the epidemiologic study of chronic disease. Unfortunately, the time from identification to application of risk reduction measures has typically been delayed by as long as decades (e.g., Pap smears for cervical cancer, mammography for breast cancer, and smoking cessation for lung cancer prevention). The slow growth of prostate cancer might allow an extended window of opportunity for early detection and intervention.

Historically, the meticulously collected and archived records of the Church of Jesus Christ of the Latter Day Saints (Mormons) in Utah have contributed to awareness and investigation of documented family clusters of diseases, including prostate cancer (Ekman, 1999). Additionally, in an article regarding familial clustering of prostate cancer, Wolfe (1960) indicated the risk is three times higher for a relative of a prostate cancer patient to acquire the disease himself. The modern era of epidemiological study began in the early 1980s when several publications reported on the association between prostate cancer and family history (Bishop & Skolnick, 1984). In 1982, Meikle and Stanish reported the higher risk for brothers to contract prostate cancer as opposed to their brothers-in-law who lived under similar environmental conditions.

The number of large scale studies of prostate cancer in the past may have been limited by technical difficulties in measuring endocrine function, especially during the time when prostate cancer is present but not yet symptomatic. While the etiology and risk factors for prostate cancer are not yet completely understood, several elements are consistently associated with an increased risk of developing this disease. Only age, race, and family history are known risk factors. However, the interest in prostate cancer has grown substantially in recent decades and much progress has been made in the investigation of contributing risk factors and biomarkers for this disease. Because prostate cancer is a potentially curable disease when diagnosed at an early stage, recent research has focused on early detection and identification of these risk factors. Furthermore, the dramatic increase in the number of prostate cancer cases and the steady increase in mortality (that has only recently begun to decline) has placed the present focus on identification and prevention of risk factors and risk reduction.

REVIEW OF MAJOR STUDIES, RESEARCHERS, AND METHODOLOGY

Age

Prostate cancer is primarily a disease of aging; the incidence rises faster with age than any other malignancy (Haas & Sakr, 1997). More than

80% of prostate cancers are diagnosed in men 65 years of age or older. It is well established that African American men have higher rates of prostate cancer than White males. The median age at diagnosis for a White male is 71 years and for an African American male is 69 years (Fowler & Bigler, 1999).

Clinically significant (i.e., symptomatic) prostate cancer is rare in men under the age of 40. With each succeeding decade of life after 40, a man's risk of developing the disease increases. Autopsy studies of men who died of causes other than prostate cancer have suggested that as many as 60 to 70% of men over the age of 80 have evidence of latent prostate cancer, although the vast majority of cases will not be clinically apparent or significant (Doherty & Breslin, 1996). Numerous genetic alterations resulting from cumulative damage to DNA over the course of a man's life may partially explain this higher incidence. An increase in the elderly population because of longer life expectancy will lead to the continuation of prostate cancer as a major health concern.

Race

Black men in the United States have the highest incidence of prostate cancer in the world; prostate cancer is nearly twice as common among African American men as it is among White American men (Brawley, Knopf, & Thompson, 1998). Black men have a mortality rate of 55.1/100,000 compared to 24.7/100,000 for White men (Aronson & Freeland, 2000). Blacks tend to be seen by physicians when the cancer is at a more advanced stage and thus have worse outcomes than Whites. Prostate cancer also develops earlier in the lives of African American men, who are twice as likely as White men to get the disease when they are still in their early fifties (Bostwick, MacLennan, & Larson, 1999).

Hormonal factors have been proposed as a possible explanation for racial variation in prostate cancer. African American men have a 13% higher level of bioavailable testosterone than do White men, and they appear to be exposed to higher levels of estrogen and testosterone in utero (Giovannucci, 1996). Fowler and Bigler (1999) prospectively studied a large group of Veteran's Administration patients and found that the mean prostate specific antigen (PSA) concentration for Blacks was much higher than for Whites. African American men may also have a higher incidence of mutations in a prostate cancer susceptibility gene. A familial predisposition syndrome for prostate cancer (e.g., hereditary prostate cancer, or HPC 1) has been found to be more prevalent in African Americans than in White Americans (Cooney et al., 1997). A number of genetic, social, dietary and other environmental factors have also been proposed to explain racial differences. Smith and colleagues performed a large scale screening study which confirmed the higher prevalence and advanced stage of prostate cancer in Black men; however, they also reached the conclusion that African American men had a lower compliance rate for getting biopsies and for undergoing radical surgery than did White men (Smith, Bullock, Catalona, & Herschman, 1996). Socioeconomic factors such as differences in attitudes toward health care, variances in health care access, willingness to participate in the selection of treatment modality, and subsequent commitment to follow through with treatment recommendations are all factors that could ultimately explain some of the racial differences or confound study results. However, stratification for socioeconomic and educational level was not found to negate differences in incidence and mortality in a series of other studies (Haas & Sakr, 1997).

Ethnicity

Different ethnic groups have different rates of clinically detectable prostate cancer. Native Americans, Mexican and Chinese Americans have lower rates than Americans whose ancestors came from Northern Europe. Globally, the rate of prostate cancer is highest in North America and northwestern Europe; Japan and other parts of Asia have the lowest rates. It is only the rate of *clinically* apparent prostate cancer that changes from one population group to another; the rate of *microscopic* prostate cancer (determined at autopsy) is roughly the same all over the world. When men move and become indoctrinated into a new culture, they eventually assume the same risks for prostate cancer as the men who have lived in that culture all their lives. For example, two generations after Japanese men move to the United States, their risk for having clinically apparent prostate cancer approaches that of White American males (Bostwick et al., 1999). Ethnic variations in prostate cancer may be partially explained by differences in screening practices as well as environmental influences.

Family History

Familial risk factors play a significant role in the development of prostate cancer. Overall, about 9% of all cases may be directly attributed to a family history, although this has been reported to be as high as 43% among men younger than 55 years of age (Giovannucci, 1996). Members of families with a high incidence of prostate cancer may be at an increased risk either because of shared environmental exposure or similar genetic make-up. Early reports of a familial influence on risk for prostate cancer were substantiated in the Utah Genealogic database

(Giovannucci, 1995). The disease is familial if two family members are diagnosed with prostate cancer. Approximately 25% of all men have a known family history of prostate cancer (Villineuve, Johnson, Kreiger, Maa, & The Canadian Cancer Registries Epidemiological Risk Group, 1999). The risk of prostate cancer increases with the numbers of affected first-degree relatives. A man with one affected first-degree relative is estimated to have a two- to three-fold greater risk of prostate cancer than the general population (Zlotta & Schulman, 1998). The risk for a man with both a first degree and a second degree relative who have prostate cancer may be increased by a factor of six above the general population. When diagnosed, it is usually discovered at a younger age and is often more aggressive (Doherty & Breslin, 1996). The potential role of endogenous hormones as the underlying etiology of familial prostate cancer warrants further study.

Heredity

It is important to distinguish between hereditary and familial prostate cancers. Genetic factors are particularly important at younger ages and the attributable risk of strong genetic factors could be as high as 43% (Giovannucci, 1996). True hereditary disorders were first distinguished from familial clusters through the use of segregation analysis in 1992 (Carter, Beaty, Steinberg, Childs, & Walsh). Heredity, specifically an autosomal dominant, Mendelian inheritance pattern of a rare, highly penetrant high-risk allele, is thought to be responsible for approximately 9% of prostate cancers. A major prostate cancer susceptibility locus was recently discovered to be located on chromosome 1 (1q 24-25) by Swedish and American scientists (Cooney et al., 1997). This hereditary prostate cancer gene, called HPC1, predisposes men to develop prostate cancer and is believed to be involved in 33% of hereditary prostate cancers, or 3% of all cases. Studies have shown that cancers linked to this gene occur earlier in life, are of a higher grade and stage than other types, and are more prevalent in African American men than Caucasian American men. Preliminary research on HPC2, HPCX (found on X chromosome) and CAPB (cancers of prostate and brain) is under way, and genetic tests are not yet available (American Cancer Society, 2000). Other loci at 1q 42.2-43 and 8p 22.1 have also been identified as possible major susceptibility genes.

Similarly, gene mutations identified as predisposing factors of breast cancer, specifically BRCA1 and BRCA2 genes, have been implicated to confer an increased risk of prostate cancer (Ekman, 1999) as have variations in certain gene lengths. Variants of the Vitamin D receptor (VDR) gene appear to increase risk of prostate cancer in African Americans. The number of trinucliotide repeats (CAG) or sequences (GGN) are also felt to be associated with high grade or advanced stages. Confirmatory studies are being performed (Brawley et al., 1998).

Dietary Factors

Nutritional factors have long been implicated as risk factors in the development of prostate cancer. Food may either alter hormonal balance, be metabolized to a carcinogen, or contain vitamins or nutrients that are protective against prostate cancer.

Fat consumption is likely the most studied dietary link to the risk of developing prostate cancer (Ekman, 1999). Although the data are inconsistent, there is strong support for an association between high intake of animal fat and prostate cancer risk (Brawley et al., 1998). Some experts suggest that a high-fat diet approximately doubles the risk of prostate cancer (Giovannucci, 1996; Mills, 1999). The specific type of fat or groups of fatty acids may also affect risk.

Men who follow high-fat (particularly fat from red meats), low-fiber diets appear to have an increased incidence of prostate cancer; conversely, a low-fat, high-fiber diet is associated with a lower risk. This may explain, in part, why the incidence of clinically significant prostate cancer is low in Asian men, who typically consume low-fat diets, and high in European and North American men who typically consume high-fat diets (Doherty & Breslin, 1996).

One proposed explanation for this association is that a high-fat intake has been associated with increased levels of serum testosterone, and higher circulating levels of androgens are associated with an increase in prostate cancer incidence (Chan, Stampfer, & Giovannucci, 1998). Vegetarian and high-fiber diets are associated with lower testosterone and estradiol levels because fiber, when excreted in the feces, lowers plasma levels by binding to sex steroids (Haas & Sakr, 1997).

A second possible explanation for this association is that a high-fat diet increases levels of *insulin-like growth factor (IGF-1)* which plays an important role in both cell proliferation and carcinogenesis. IGF-1 is a mitogen for prostate epithelial cells. A strong positive association has been observed between IGF-1 levels and prostate cancer risk, independent of baseline PSA levels (Chan et al., 1998). The American Cancer Society (ACS) reports that men with high levels of IGF-1 are more than four times as likely to contract prostate cancer than those without the growth factor (Bostwick et al., 1999).

Another weakly supported theory is that heterocyclic amines, mutagens formed during the cooking of meat, may contribute to increased risk of prostate cancer. Well-done meat has been associated with increased risk of colorectal and breast cancers. There was an especially high risk of prostate cancer observed in men who ate well-done beefsteak (Norrish et al., 1999).

Diets high in beta-carotene—fruits, yellow and green vegetables, beans, peas, lentils, and cereals—have all been associated with lower prostate cancer mortality, but study results have been inconsistent, and clear associations have not yet been established. Beta-carotene is a natural substance found in fruits and vegetables that the body converts to Vitamin A. Vitamin A has been shown to inhibit the growth of cancer cells. In a population-based, case-control study in New Zealand during 1996 to 1997 the dietary intake of beta-carotene was found to be largely unassociated with prostate cancer risk (Norrish, Jackson, Sharpe, & Skeaff, 2000).

Much attention has been focused on the protective effects of *lycopenes,* a substance found in tomatoes, against the development of prostate cancer. Lycopene, the predominant carotenoid in the prostate gland, acts as an antioxidant. Intake of tomatoes or tomato-based products was found to be strongly related to decreased risk of prostate cancer in several studies (Giovannuci, 1995; Mills, Beeson, Phillips, & Fraser, 1989). The inverse relationship between lycopenes and the development of prostate cancer was found to be particularly apparent for more aggressive cancers and in men who do not consume sources of beta-carotene. In a 1982 prospective case-control study using plasma samples obtained for the Physicians' Health Study, lycopene was the only antioxidant found to show a statistically significant inverse relationship with prostate cancer (Gann et al., 1999). This study controlled for age, smoking, body-mass index (BMI), exercise, alcohol, multivitamin use, and plasma cholesterol level.

Cohen, Kristal, and Stanford (2000) studied the association of fruit and vegetable intake with prostate cancer in a population-based, case-controlled study of over 1,200 men under the age of 65 who lived in the Seattle area from 1993 to 1996. Although no association was found between fruit intake (including lycopenes) and prostate cancer risk, results suggested that high consumption of vegetables (especially cruciferous vegetables) was associated with reduced risk of prostate cancer.

Results of studies regarding the influence of fat and other dietary influences on prostate cancer risk are inconsistent. For example, results from the Canadian National Enhanced Cancer Surveillance System found that total fat consumption and tomato intake were not associated with prostate cancer. This large study included over 3,200 subjects in a population-based, case-control study conducted in 8 of 10 Canadian provinces between 1994 and 1997 (Villeneuve et al., 1999).

Occupational and Environmental Exposure

A man's risk may be influenced by where he lives or works. Prostate cancer rates are highest in the areas of the world which get the least amount of *sun*. In the United States, rates are highest in the northeastern states of New England and lowest in the Sunbelt states. Some evidence suggests that prostate cancer rates are higher in men who have low *Vitamin D* levels. Sunlight is a major factor in Vitamin D production because ultra-violet radiation from the sun stimulates the body to manufacture Vitamin D in the skin. It has been postulated that Vitamin D, which appears to inhibit the growth of tumors, somehow prevents microscopic prostate cancer from progressing (Bostwick et al., 1999). In yet another study, men who lived in rural settings were found to have higher stages of prostate cancer than men who lived in urban areas (Haas & Sakr, 1997). This hypothesis appears to contradict the theory that increased sun exposure results in lower rates of prostate cancer.

No occupation has been firmly identified as a risk factor for prostate cancer despite a large number of studies performed on the subject. The areas of occupation best studied are *farming, cadmium* exposure, and *rubber manufacturing* (Giovannucci, 1996).

A review of the literature on the possible link between farming and prostate cancer reported a positive association (10 of which were statistically significant) in 17 of 24 reported studies (Blair & Zahn, 1991). However, in addition to increased sun exposure, farmers are also exposed to other risks such as herbicides, pesticides and fertilizers which may also increase their risks (Ekman, 1999). The adverse effects of potentially hazardous carcinogens such as pesticides and herbicides used by farmers and agricultural workers on their prostate cancer mortality have not been consistently reported in the literature.

Environmental exposure to cadmium, a nonessential trace mineral, appears to slightly increase a man's risk of developing the disease. Cadmium is a trace mineral that interferes with Vitamin D synthesis, a Vitamin D antagonist that directly replaces zinc. The prostate gland has the highest concentration of zinc of all body organs. Zinc is responsible for a number of intra-prostate functions such as DNA and RNA repair. Workers involved in farming, welding, and electroplating are particularly at risk for exposure to cadmium (Doherty & Breslin, 1996). Studies linking cadmium to prostate cancer risk are suggestive but inconclusive.

Data to establish a causal association between prostate cancer and exposure within the rubber industry are conflicting and inconclusive. A review by the International Agency for Research on Cancer in 1982 concluded that there was no causal association between prostate cancer and any specific exposure to carcinogenic compounds or solvents used within the rubber industry.

Job-related *physical activity* has shown a modest inverse relationship with prostate cancer but the data, once again, are inconsistent. Physically active and aerobically trained men have reduced levels of circulating testosterone compared to sedentary men (Villeneuve et al., 1999). Eleven studies that evaluated the effect of physical activity and prostate cancer were reviewed by Kiningham in 1998. He identified an inverse relationship between physical activity and a risk factor for prostate cancer. Specifically, strenuous occupational activity at younger ages appeared to be protective (Villeneuve et al., 1999).

Hormones

Studies of the role of hormonal influence on the pathophysiology of prostate cancer are compelling, however, no consistent linkage has been formed. The male hormone *testosterone* appears to be an essential factor in prostate cancer. Androgens promote cell proliferation and inhibit cell death, and exogenous testosterone is thought to increase human prostate cancer risk (Brawley et al., 1998). The testicles produce and secrete the body's main source of testosterone. Studies find that men whose testicles were damaged or removed before puberty almost never develop prostate cancer (Chan et al., 1998). For more information on the role of hormones in prostate development, see chapter 8. Evidence is accumulating that suggests that androgenic stimulation over a prolonged period of time is a promoter of prostate cancer (Brawley et al., 1998). Lab tests have shown that prostate cancer can be induced in rats by giving them testosterone for long periods of time (Chan et al., 1998).

The value of serum hormone measurement to identify higher risk groups for prostate cancer or benign prostatic hyperplasia (BPH) is an area of continuing uncertainty (Montie & Pienta, 1994). The relationship between *BPH* and prostate cancer is not well-established although both are common in aging men and both are androgen-dependent (Monty & Pienta, 1994). BPH is a non-cancerous enlargement of the prostate gland that may interfere with initiating or stopping urinary flow. It is possible that BPH does not increase risk of developing prostate cancer, but increases the opportunity of being diagnosed with prostate cancer. BPH and prostate cancer are often diagnosed concurrently, although in different parts of the gland.

High-grade *prostatic intraepithelial neoplasia (PIN)* is now an accepted term for the preinvasive stage of adenocarcinoma (Bostwick et al., 1999). Most studies suggest that patients with PIN will develop carcinoma within 10 years. Androgen deprivation therapy decreases the prevalence and extent of PIN, making anti-androgen therapy a potential form of chemoprevention.

The literature contains some reports that link prostate cancer to an active *sexual life*. Early sexual experiences, venereal disease (especially involving the human papilloma virus), and multiple sexual partners before marriage are also weakly linked to an increased risk of acquiring prostate cancer (Haas & Sakr, 1997).

Vasectomy has been studied in case control and cohort studies and shown to have a slightly increased risk for developing prostate cancer, but findings are inconsistent and available data are insufficient to confirm this hypothesis (Giovannucci, 1995). The risk is reported to be higher in men under the age of 35 at the time of vasectomy, and the risk is suspected to increase cumulatively during the time following vasectomy (Giovannucci, 1995). These findings may be explained in part by the higher level of health-seeking behaviors demonstrated by men who seek vasectomy, and who are, therefore, more likely to be screened for the early detection of prostate cancer. A report of two large cohort studies published in 1993 revealed a 50% increased risk of prostate cancer associated with having had a vasectomy (Giovannucci et al., 1993). The authors propose that vasectomy may increase serum testosterone levels, antisperm antibodies, or immunologic reaction, or create an imbalance in growth hormones or their inhibitors (Haas & Sakr, 1997). To the contrary, other reports conclude that a hormonal mechanism is not known, since plasma testosterone is either unaltered or only modestly changed after vasectomy. Most recent studies have not found any increased risk among men who have had this operation; any risk, if it exists, is small (Brawley et al., 1998).

Miscellaneous

The scientific literature regarding a link between *cigarette smoking* and prostate cancer is also conflicting. The risk of prostate cancer was inversely related to the number of cigarettes smoked daily, but the number of cumulative "pack years" (i.e., packs per day multiplied by the number of years smoked) or the number of years since smoking cessation occurred were not found to be related to the development of prostate cancer (Lund-Nilsen, Johnson, & Vatten, 2000). It has been reported that cigarette smoking may increase the development of prostate cancer by elevating levels of testosterone. On the other hand, carcinogenic components of cigarette smoke have also been recognized as factors that may increase the overall risk of prostate cancer. It has been proposed that the increased risk of prostate cancer among smokers may be influenced by other high-risk health care and lifestyle behaviors in this population.

For the most part, epidemiological studies have not supported an association between BMI, *obesity*, and an increased risk of prostate cancer. Taller individuals have a higher risk of developing several malignancies, including breast and colon cancers (Albanes & Taylor, 1990), but data for prostate cancer risk are conflicting. Attained *height* and childhood obesity may reflect hormonal events during puberty and adolescence which are characterized by changes in sex hormone levels, growth hormones, and IGF-1 (Chan, Stampfer, & Giovannucci, 1998; Giovannucci, Rimm, Stampfer, Colditz, & Willett, 1997). A large retrospective cohort study of data collected from 135,000 male construction workers between 1971 and 1975 concluded that various aspects of body size, especially high body mass index, were related to an excessive risk of death from prostate cancer (Andersson et al., 1997).

Following much study, *alcohol* consumption has not been firmly linked with prostate cancer. A review of studies conducted over a 25-year span by Breslow and Weed (1998) found no convincing support for an association between prostate cancer and moderate drinking, and limited evidence of increased risk associated with heavy drinking. Results of a meta-analysis of six cohort and 27 case-control studies published before July, 1998 concluded that there was no association between prostate cancer and alcohol consumption (Dennis, 2000).

Future Directions: Chemoprevention

The high incidence and mortality associated with prostate cancer, coupled with the failure of conventional chemotherapy, radiation therapy, and surgical interventions to effectively control the disease compels us to seek and develop innovative ways to combat this disease. In prostate cancer, the time from tumor initiation until clinical detection usually covers a period of decades, presenting an opportune time to interrupt the process of carcinogenesis with the use of chemoprevention agents. The most important rationale for hormonal chemoprevention of prostate cancer has been the realization that prostate cancer does not develop in men castrated before puberty (Chan et al., 1998). Although programs utilizing PSA screening have resulted in diagnosis at an earlier stage of disease and have greatly reduced the incidence of metastatic disease at time of initial diagnosis, there is no direct evidence that screening with early detection has resulted in improved survival. Chemoprevention refers to the use of either natural or synthetic chemical substances to prevent induction of a malignancy or to inhibit, reverse, or delay its promotion or progression. Chemoprevention is an alternative approach to prevent, delay, or stop the development of cancer in high risk individuals. Healthy individuals at high risk for prostate cancer or who have a precancerous condition, or wish to prevent a recurrence or development of a second primary tumor might be appropriate candidates for chemoprevention studies (Swan & Ford, 1997).

The *Prostate Cancer Prevention Trial (PCPT)*, started in 1993, is an NCI-funded multicenter, double-blinded, randomized, placebo-controlled trial. It was created to determine if finasteride (Proscar®) could prevent the development of early prostate cancer in men at risk of developing the disease based on age, family history, or history of BPH. The study enrolled 18,882 men over the age of 55 years with normal digital rectal exam (DRE) and a PSA < 3. The primary endpoint of the study is the occurrence of biopsy-proven prostate cancer of any stage or grade (Krishnan, Ruffin & Brenner, 1998).

The study design called for a three-month placebo period during which subject compliance was assessed. Once deemed acceptable, the subjects were randomized to receive either finasteride, 5 mg daily, or a placebo for a period of seven years. DRE and PSA are performed annually; if DRE is found to be abnormal, prostate biopsy is performed. For subjects in the placebo arm, a PSA > 4 ng/ml warrants biopsy. Following completion of treatment, all subjects undergo prostate biopsy. Quality of life, dietary and life style questionnaires are also being collected. A secondary hypothesis of the study is that treatment with finasteride will prevent development of BPH.

Finasteride, an inhibitor of the enzyme 5-alpha reductase, may prevent prostate cancer by decreasing androgen stimulation of the prostate gland. Five-alpha reductase is necessary to convert testosterone to dihydrotestosterone (DHT), the major androgenic compound in the gland. Finasteride also lowers prostatic volume and improves urinary flow. Serum testosterone levels are not affected and levels of PSA are known to be lowered by 50% in men taking finasteride (Montironi, Mazzucchelli, Marshall, & Bartels, 1999). The side-effect profile of finasteride reveals it to be extremely well tolerated and nontoxic. Impotence and decreased ejaculatory volume were the most frequently reported side effects with a 4% incidence, and decreased libido occurred in 3%. Dizziness, headache, breast pain, dysuria, testicular pain, eye changes, rash, facial swelling, and gynecomastia are uncommon side effects.

Scientists at the NCI Division of Cancer Prevention and Control, in conjunction with the Southwest Oncology Group and Intergroup participants, are presently preparing for the largest prostate cancer study ever conducted. *The Selenium and Vitamin E Chemoprevention Trial* (SELECT), a phase III double-blind, placebo-controlled study, hypothesizes that prostate cancer may be prevented by Vitamin E alone or through a combination of Vitamin E and selenium. The rationale for using selenium and Vitamin E as chemopreventive agents grows out of the substances' roles as antioxidants. Selenium is thought to be synergistic with Vitamin E's antioxidant effect.

Selenium is a trace nutrient essential for enzyme activity, and has demonstrated anti-carcinogenic effects in a variety of study types (Chan et al., 1998). A trial evaluating the use of selenium for skin cancer prevention failed to establish a significant reduction in skin cancers; however, analysis of secondary end points revealed a statistically significant reduction in prostate cancer incidence (63%) in men randomized to take 200 mg daily supplements (Clark et al., 1998). This finding was supported in a second large investigation that examined high selenium levels in the toenails of men with prostate cancer. In this study, a 50% reduced risk of advanced prostate cancer was observed when compared to study controls. This study controlled for the possible confounding factors of dietary fiber, smoking, age, BMI, geographic region, family history, and prior vasectomy (Yoshizawa et al., 1998).

Similar findings have been reported among males who receive *Vitamin E*. Vitamin E functions as the major lipid soluble antioxidant that protects cell membranes from free radical damage and DNA instability. The most active form of Vitamin E is alpha-tocopherocol, which is also the most abundant and widely distributed vitamin in nature, as well as the most predominant form in human tissue. Vitamin E is present in a wide range of foods, including vegetable oils, margarine and shortening, egg yolks, milk fat, vegetables, nuts, and whole wheat products. Studies are inconsistent with regard to a decrease in association between prostate cancer and Vitamin E, but more consistent information exists regarding the association between Vitamin E with lung and colorectal cancer, where Vitamin E intake is inversely related to risk. A chemoprevention trial of 29,000 male smokers who received 50 mg daily supplements of Vitamin E demonstrated a 32% decrease in prostate cancer incidence and a 41% reduction in prostate cancer mortality when compared to placebo group (Heinonen et al., 1998). These findings have yet to be confirmed in prospective trials.

The goal of the SELECT trial is to recruit 32,400 men at 250 medical centers nationwide who are > 55 years if White, or > 50 years if African American. A lower age eligibility is specified for African American men because the incidence of prostate cancer for African American men ages 50 to 55 years old is comparable with that for Caucasian men ages 55 to 60 years old. Study duration will be 12 years, with a five-year accrual period, and a minimum of 7 years of treatment. The protocol will use a 2 x 2 factorial design that will permit simultaneous testing of both selenium and Vitamin E in order to determine whether individual or combined use is more successful in preventing or reducing the incidence of prostate cancer. A correlational study of the effects of selenium and Vitamin E on prostate carcinogenesis will also be conducted.

Difuromethylornithine (DFMO) is another potential prostate cancer chemoprevention agent which acts by inhibiting cell proliferation. DFMO has been shown to have activity in several animal tumors, including prostate cancer, in early phase clinical trials.

The ability of *retinoids* to induce differentiation led to a phase I clinical trial to assess tolerance and prostate cancer chemoprevention activity in men with a history of elevated serum PSA and negative prostate biopsies. It is doubtful that a large-scale chemoprevention trial employing retinoids will be possible due to the spectrum of serious side effects of retinoids on a study of healthy men (Brawley & Thompson, 1994).

Recent interest in herbal therapies has led to studies investigating the use of *Serenoa repens* (saw palmetto) for the treatment of symptomatic BPH and progressive prostate cancer. The fruits and extracts of the herb are used alone or in combination with other phytotherapeutic agents as an alternative medicine to improve urinary tract symptoms and urinary flow in moderately symptomatic patients with BPH. There are anecdotal reports of anti-prostate cancer activity with decline in serum PSA in patients with progressive prostate cancer. The literature is limited and further randomized and controlled trials are required to evaluate an indication for saw palmetto for prostate cancer prevention.

Economic and Ethical Concerns

The financial burden of prostate cancer is significant and is growing exponentially. Demographic trends in the next few decades reveal an increasing population of older men with higher risk for prostate cancer (Thompson, Feigl, & Coltman, 1996). Resource allocations are limited by health care expenditures and limited resources. The introduction of PSA testing has led to controversy regarding the appropriateness of screening and subsequent treatment in elderly men.

The ACS currently recommends annual DRE and PSA measurement for men older than 50 years of age (Smith, Mettlin, Davis, & Eyre, 2000). The economic benefit of early detection and treatment is mitigated by the many successive years of health care and the later costs associated with cancer progression. Coley, Barry, Fleming, Fahs, and Mulley (1997b) estimated the cost of an early detection program with DRE and PSA evaluation in three hypothetical age groups using Medicare fee schedules. The documented average number of days of life saved per person screened was 11 days for patients 50 to 59 years, 7 days for patients 60 to 69 years, and 3 days for patients 70 to 79 years. The average estimated cost per person screened was $216.00, $387.00, and $532.00, respectively. Furthermore, the cost per year of life saved as a result of screening was $12,491.00, $18,769.00, and $65,909.00. Coley and colleagues (1997b) conclude that DRE and PSA measurement is cost-effective only for men in their 50s and 60s, and that available evidence does not justify current ACS guidelines because the average health benefit is no more than a few additional weeks of life expectancy. Albertsen (1996) concurs that the costs of implementing a screening program are enormous, and the overall benefit to a population of men screened for prostate cancer can be measured in days of additional life gained, rather than in months or years.

A major acceleration in prostate cancer research funding by the National Institutes of Health began in 1999 with funding of $180 million, a 60% increase over 1998 funding of $114 million. The Prostate Cancer Review Group report completed in 1998 identifies $420 million worth of potential research opportunities that could be supported in the year 2003 (Varnus, 1999). The National Cancer Institute's budget for prostate cancer has also risen considerably in recent years.

Relationships to Nursing Practice

Nurses are in a position of vulnerability as to whether they should recommend screening for elderly, asymptomatic men since the recommendations and policies of leading medical and cancer organizations are contradictory. Individualized counseling, education, and risk assessment along with involvement of patients and spouses in the decision of whether to screen for prostate cancer in asymptomatic elderly men will guide the oncology nurse in making recommendations.

The role of nurses as patient advocates has become increasingly important due to diminished health care resources and managed care constraints. Nurses play an important role in prostate cancer risk assessment and screening, patient, family, and public education regarding risk-reduction strategies, and through involvement in conducting research and disseminating clinical research findings. Nurses serve as an intermediary to link patients, families, and communities to cancer prevention and detection programs. Nurses must act as change agents, coordinators and directors as well as interventionists (Morra, 2000).

Scientific evidence is as important to cancer control and prevention as it is to cancer treatment. To achieve success in cancer prevention and early detection, nurses need to acknowledge the complexity of health-related behaviors and focus on improving patients' fundamental knowledge base. They must use evidence-based data as a basis for promoting informed decision making regarding lifestyle changes and participation in screening and surveillance efforts.

A quasi-experimental nursing study was performed in South Carolina to document the importance of providing educational programs as a means to increasing participation in prostate cancer screening. Recruitment was aimed toward African American men in South Carolina; subjects included 319 men without a previous history of prostate cancer, 82% of whom were African American. The authors concluded that prostate cancer knowledge was a predictor for screening participation. They further recommend that nurses specifically target African American men, who have the highest incidence of and mortality from prostate cancer (Weinrich, Weinrich, Boyd, & Atkinson, 1998).

In another nursing study of 1,432 men in South Carolina, barriers were identified which were significant predictors of nonparticipation in free prostate cancer screenings. Based on the Health Belief Model, their study hypothesized that the likelihood of participating in prostate cancer screening is determined by each man's perceived benefits minus his perceived barriers. The results of the study found (when the two main barriers of cost and lack of knowledge were eliminated) the following barriers were significant in predicting participation in prostate cancer screening: "didn't know what kind of doctor to see," "doctor's office hours were not convenient," "put it off," "didn't know where to go," and "refuse to go" (Weinrich, Reynolds, Tingen, & Starr, 2000). Dissemination of information by nurses can rectify these barriers, and possibly reduce ethnic, educational, and regional disparities in prostate cancer risk, incidence, and mortality.

Behavioral change strategies must be studied scientifically, and their selection must be based on careful analysis of efficacy within the targeted population. More research is needed to focus on the effect of socioeconomic, ethnic, and racial influences. Underserved and socioeconomically deprived populations often have the highest burden of cancer risk and mortality rate due to limited health care access, lack of insurance, unemployment, homelessness, nutrition, and transportation issues.

Successful increases in mammography rates were achieved through provider-prompting interventions, systems and policy changes (including financial support), written and verbal counseling, media-based initiatives, and community health interventions. The tremendous efforts that nursing has contributed to promoting early detection of breast cancer have resulted in increased survival for thousands of women. The same practical techniques could be applied to prostate cancer risk reduction and screening. For example, nurses can play a hands-on role in planning and coordinating health fairs and screening projects. A number of approaches to cancer screening are available, including individual screening, mass screening, case-finding, genetic testing, and work-site surveillance (Mahon, 2000).

Identification of genes involved in prostate cancer will provide new methods for prevention of this disease. Once legitimate prevention strategies are determined, nurses will have an integral role in public and individual education regarding genetic predisposition and testing. Nurses need to have a commanding knowledge of media access, infomatics, and other newer resources for communication in order to direct patients to reliable sources of information.

Basic behavioral research may contribute to the development of methods used to educate the general public about risk reduction strategies and how to prevent or change maladaptive behaviors. Nurses are in a prime position to develop decision-making aids and instruments to promote appropriate self-care and health-seeking behaviors among their patients. Other tasks include developing tools to assess quality of life (QOL), implementing evidence-based interventions to enhance QOL, evaluating health outcomes and intervening to effect change conducive to improved health.

Nurses who specialize in research may be involved in the coordination of all stages of prostate cancer clinical research. Identification of patients for participation in trials can be achieved through chart reviews and patient assessments. Nurses frequently prepare the consent forms for institutional review board submission and ensure that the patient understands the proposed treatment plan, risks and benefits of the study, and available alternatives. During the study phase, the nurse may be responsible for evaluation, grading, and documentation of toxicities. To support men who have potential risks for developing prostate cancer, nurses must offer information that may or may not be welcome or easy for them to accept. Providing information and support to help men deal with side effects and validation of concerns requires sensitivity, knowledge, and compassion.

Lack of financial support by Medicare and managed care plans to cover prevention and early detection deters many patients from participating in screening programs. The nurse must balance and protect the economic and ethical interests of the patient. A major ethical concern is related to the recommendation for prostate cancer screening in elderly men with less than a 10- to 15-year life expectancy. Some current organizational guidelines (e.g., American College of Surgeons, Agency for Health Policy and Research, American Academy of Family Physicians) eliminate screening of these older men. Gerard and Frank-Stromborg (1998) concluded that public policy should include shared decision making as a basis for a man's decision to be screened until a uniform national/international recommendation is declared for detection of early prostate cancer.

SUMMARY

To understand and participate in cancer prevention strategies the nurse will need to have a solid background in behavioral change theories, cancer pathophysiology, genetics, ethics, health care policy, educational theory, psychology, and occupational and environmental health.

The most successful approach in the goal to control cancer may well lie in prevention. Diet and lifestyle modification, elimination of occupational and environmental risks, and early diagnosis is critical in the quest to reduce the morbidity and mortality of prostate cancer. The tremendous impact of prostate cancer and the financial burden of the disease on both individuals and society has led to an increased interest in primary and secondary prevention. As the number of men at risk for developing prostate cancer grows, there will be opportunities for nurses to be more effective in their contributions toward controlling this disease. The challenge of better understanding the risk factors and using risk reduction measures will continue as we confirm new research theories and implement recommendations into practice. It is reasonable to hope that, in the near future, we will be able to identify men at risk of developing prostate cancer and better inform them about effective prevention strategies.

3

Assessment, Screening and Diagnosis of Prostate Cancer

Eun-Hyun Lee

The sobering statistics surrounding the increased incidence and prevalence of prostate cancer have compelled nurses to attend to the early detection of the disease. To do so, nurses must have a current knowledge of prostate cancer. With the information contained herein, nurses will be better prepared to assess the disease and recommend appropriate treatment to decrease the morbidity and mortality of prostate cancer.

ASSESSMENT

Symptom Pattern

The prostate is a gland located deep in the male pelvis and surrounds the proximal end of the urethra. The base of the prostate adjoins the base of the bladder (referred to as the bladder neck). The prostate is composed of three zones: the transitional zone (periurethral zone), the central zone, and the peripheral zone. Most prostate cancers arise in the peripheral zone, which is the outermost part of the gland (Vetrosky & White, 1998). Since the majority of prostate cancer arises in the peripheral zone of the gland, distant from the urethra, prostate cancer is usually asymptomatic in its early stage.

The presence of symptoms, as a result of prostate cancer, usually suggests a locally advanced or metastatic disease. Growth of prostate cancer into the urethra or bladder neck may produce obstructed bladder outlet signs and symptoms, such as an increase in urinary frequency, hesitancy, nocturia, decreased force of urinary stream, urgency, intermittency, and residuals. Local progression of the disease and obstruction of the ejaculatory ducts can result in hematospermia and decreased ejaculation volume. Uncommonly, impotence or decrease in the firmness of penile erections for intercourse may be present (Garnick, 1993; Snyder, 2000). As the tumor progresses, it commonly metastasizes to pelvic lymph nodes, bones, or visceral organs (Held-Warmkessel, 2000; Wood & Lockhart, 2000).

Pelvic lymph node invasion produces lower extremity edema or weakness, and bone metastases presents as pain in the back, hips, thighs, ribs, or shoulders. Metastatic involvement of the visceral organs, such as lungs, liver, adrenal glands, and kidneys, tends to occur late in the course of the disease. Signs related to the spread of disease include anemia, weight loss, and hematuria (if the bladder or urethra is invaded).

Nurses should assess these signs and symptoms (Table 3.1). However, it should be considered that the signs and symptoms are also indicators of other urogenital problems common in this age group, such as benign prostatic hypertrophy (BPH) or urinary track infections.

Prostate-Specific Antigen Test (PSA)

The PSA test measures the level of prostate specific antigen in the blood. PSA is a serine protease produced by the prostatic epithelial cells in the male. It is concentrated in prostatic tissue normally found in low levels in serum (Carter & Partin, 1998). Generally, the normal range of serum PSA using the most commonly used assay, Tandem®-R (Hybriteck, San Diego, CA) is from 0 to 4 ng/ml. Serum PSA levels from 4 to 10 ng/ml may be termed borderline and those above 10 ng/ml are considered high (Wood & Lockhart, 2000).

Serum PSA is not cancer specific, but prostate specific. Thus, serum PSA may rise in the presence of prostate cancer, but also in other conditions. Elevated serum PSA may be present in other nonmalignancies, such as prostatitis, and benign prostatic hypertrophy. It may also occur with mechanical manipulation of the prostate, such as a biopsy, transurethral resection of the prostate, and catheterization (Held-Warmkessel, 2000). Such false-positive test results (PSA level is elevated, but no cancer is actually present) may lead to additional medical procedures, such as guided biopsy, increased financial costs, and anxiety for men and their families (Brawer, 1999).

To enhance the sensitivity and specificity of PSA to detect prostate cancer, several PSA techniques have been proposed: age-specific PSA, PSA density, PSA velocity, and free-to-total PSA ratio. As men age, their prostate enlarges; thus, higher serum PSA levels would be expected in older men. In a prospective and community-based study with 2,119 healthy men, Oesterling and his colleagues (1993) examined the influence

TABLE 3.1 Questions Assessing Urinary Signs and Symptoms Associated with Prostate Cancer

Sign and Symptom	Assessment
Dysuria	Does the patient have difficulty initiating urination? If so, how often?
	Does the patient have difficulty maintaining or ending the urine stream?
	Does the patient need to apply pressure to the bladder to initiate urination?
	Does dribbling occur at the end of urination?
	Is there pain during urination? If so, what kind of pain? Does it persist or is it intermittent?
	Are there bladder spasms?
Frequency	How often does the patient need to urinate?
	What is the volume of each voiding?
	Does the patient void and then need to void again a few minutes later?
	Is there a reduction in the urine volume produced?
Nocturia	How many times does the patient get out of bed each night to urinate?
	Is there incontinence at night?
Hematuria	Is there blood in the urine? Clots?
	What is the color of the urine?
Other	Does the urine have an odor?
	Is particulate matter present in the urine?
	When did the patient void most recently?
	Can the patient feel his bladder through the abdominal wall?
	Is there flank pain?
	How many urinary tract infections has the patient had in the last 12 months?
	Has there been a change in the strength of penile erections?

Note. From: Black, J. & Matassarin-Jacobs, E (Eds.). *Luckmann & Sorensen's medical-surgical nursing: A psychophysiologic approach* (4th ed.). Philadelphia: Saunders.

of age and prostatic size on the serum PSA. Age and prostate size were significantly correlated with serum PSA ($r = .43$, $p < .0001$; $r = .55$, $p < .0001$, respectively). Age and prostatic size were also correlated ($r = .25$, $p < .0001$). The investigators noted that PSA should be interpreted in relation to age-specific references, rather than rely on a single reference range for men of all age groups. They recommended the following age-specific reference range for serum PSA for men in various age groups:

1. 40–49 years is 0.0–2.5 ng/ml;
2. 50–59 years, 0.0–3.5 ng/ml;
3. 60–69 years, 0.0 to 4.5 ng/ml; and
4. 70–79 years, 0.0–6.5 ng/ml.

Race is considered to be an important factor in setting age-specific PSA reference ranges. In a study of 3,475 military men (1802 White, 1673 African American) aged 40 to 79 years, Morgan and colleagues (1996) investigated age- and race-specific reference ranges to determine PSA ranges (see Table 3.2).

PSA density (PSAD) is a measure to enhance PSA specificity by adjusting the PSA level for prostate volume. PSAD is calculated by dividing the serum PSA level by the transrectal ultrasound (TRUS)-determined volume of the prostate. A higher PSAD indicates a greater likelihood of cancer. However, there is a discrepancy in the efficacy of PSAD in prostate cancer detection. Some studies demonstrated an enhanced efficacy of PSAD over PSA alone to predict the presence of prostate cancer (Bazinet et al., 1994; Benson, Whang, Olsson, McMahon, & Cooner, 1992). Others reported that PSAD offered no improvement over PSA alone in men undergoing prostate biopsy (Brawer, Arambura, Chen, Preston, & Ellis, 1993; Mettlin et al., 1994). The possible reason for the discrepancy might be inaccurate prostate volume calculations and a lack of reproducibility on a transrectal ultrasound (Frydenberg, Stricker, & Kaye, 1997). Although PSAD is not a perfect predictor of cancer, a PSAD of 0.15 or greater is used for counseling men with intermediate PSA levels (4.0–10.0 ng/ml) about the need for prostate biopsy (Bazinet et al., 1994).

PSA velocity (PSAV) refers to the amount that PSA levels increase over time. Carter and his colleagues (1992), who first introduced this method, found that a PSAV of 0.75 ng/ml or greater in a one-year period might be suggestive of the presence of prostate cancer. It is important to note that normal activities (e.g., exercise, sexual activity) may alter serum PSA estimations, and thereby reduce the effectiveness of PSAV (Frydenberg, Stricker, & Kaye, 1997).

PSA circulates in the blood in molecular forms, free and bound forms. The free-to-total PSA ratio tends to be lower in men with prostate

TABLE 3.2 Age- and Race-Specific Reference Ranges for Serum PSA

Age	Whites	African Americans
40–49	0.0–2.5 ng/ml	0.0–2.0 ng/ml
50–59	0.0–3.5 ng/ml	0.0–4.0 ng/ml
60–69	0.0–3.5 ng/ml	0.0–4.5 ng/ml
70–79	0.0–3.5 ng/ml	0.0–5.5 ng/ml

Note. From: Morgan, T. O., Jacobsen, S. J., McCarthy, W. F., Jacobson, D. J., McLeod, D. G., & Moul, J. W. (1996). Age-specific reference ranges for serum prostate-specific antigen in black men. *The New England Journal of Medicine, 335*, 304–310.

cancer than in men with benign prostatic hyperplasia (Stenman et al., 1991). Some investigators have suggested that a free-to-total PSA ratio is applicable to detect prostate cancer in men with PSA values between 4.0 and 10.0 ng/ml (Catalona et al., 1995; Vashi et al., 1997). However, more studies are needed to determine whether the free-to-total PSA ratio can be effectively used for the detection of prostate cancer.

Digital Rectal Examination

The DRE is the most widely used initial test for the diagnosis of prostate cancer. Since the prostate is located in front of the rectum, it can be palpated with a lubricated-gloved index finger through the wall of the rectum (Figure 3.1). During the examination, the size, lesions, symmetry, and texture of the prostate are assessed (Coley, Barry, & Mulley, 1997).

Although the DRE is a simple and inexpensive method of screening for prostate cancer, it has its limitations. Only posterior and lateral areas of the prostate gland can be palpated by the DRE. Therefore, the approximately 40% of cancer that occurs in the anterior to midline of the prostate cannot be detected (Littrup, Lee, & Mettlin, 1992). Another limitation is the difficulty in detecting small lesions, especially less than 1.5 cm (Lee et al., 1988).

Combined Use of DRE and PSA

Although some studies have shown that the PSA is more effective in detecting prostate cancer than the DRE (Brawer, Catalona, & McConnell, 1992; Kramer, Brown, Prorok, Potosky, & Gohagan, 1993), the most effective method for early detection of prostate cancer is the combined use of the DRE and PSA (Carter & Partin, 1998). In a prospective study, Catalona and colleagues (1994) studied the efficacy of the DRE and

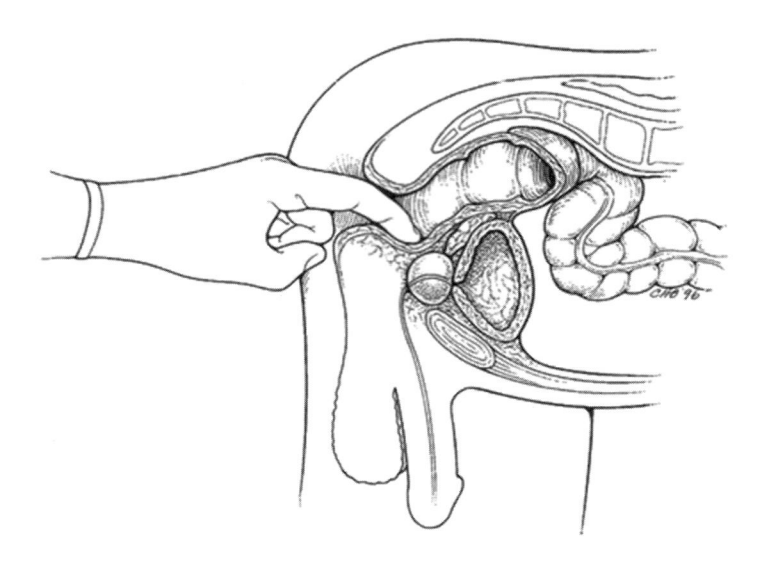

FIGURE 3.1 Digital rectal examination.
Note. From American Cancer Society (http://www3.cancer.org/cancerinfo/load_cont.asp?st=ds&ct=36).

serum PSA in 6,630 men. Biopsies were performed in patients with PSA levels greater than 4 ng/ml or a suspicious DRE. Of 1,167 biopsies performed cancer was detected in 264, resulting in a cancer detection rate that was 3.2% for the DRE, 4.6% for the PSA, and 5.8% for the DRE and PSA combined. The investigators concluded that the use of the PSA with the DRE enhances early prostate cancer detection. Figure 3.2 presents the process of early prostate cancer detection using both the DRE and PSA, as recommended by the AUA.

Transrectal Ultrasonography (TRUS)

TRUS is a commonly used method for visualization of the prostate. Its value is in the evaluation of the volume of the prostate and the detection of cancer in suspect areas (Narayan, 1995). In a study comparing the clinical usefulness of TRUS and the DRE in the detection of prostate cancer in 784 men over age 60 (Lee et al., 1988), TRUS was two times more likely to detect prostate cancer than the DRE. Based on this finding, the authors concluded that TRUS was more sensitive than the DRE in the detection of prostate cancer, and they advocated broader implementation and evaluation of TRUS as a tool for early detection.

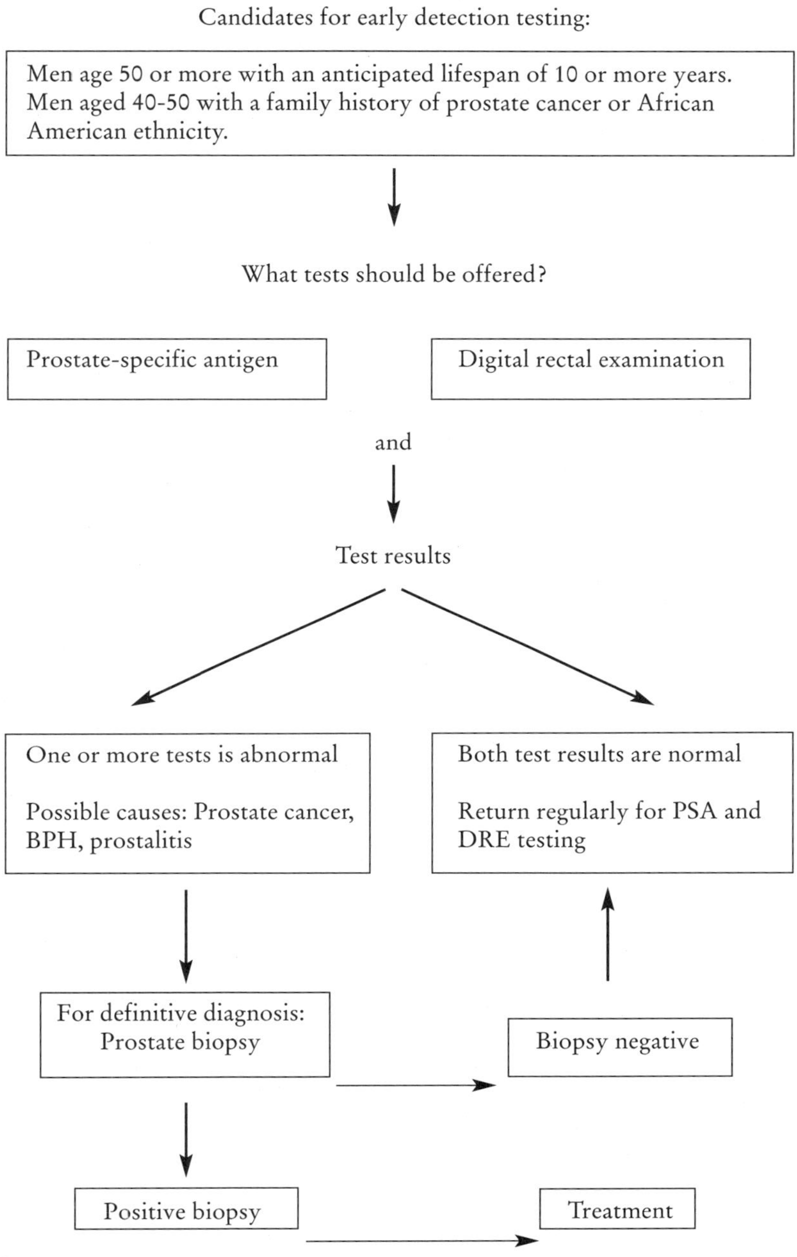

Assessment, Screening, Diagnosis 39

Candidates for early detection testing:

Men age 50 or more with an anticipated lifespan of 10 or more years. Men aged 40-50 with a family history of prostate cancer or African American ethnicity.

What tests should be offered?

Prostate-specific antigen

Digital rectal examination

and

Test results

One or more tests is abnormal

Possible causes: Prostate cancer, BPH, prostalitis

Both test results are normal

Return regularly for PSA and DRE testing

For definitive diagnosis: Prostate biopsy

Biopsy negative

Positive biopsy

Treatment

FIGURE 3.2 Early detection of prostate cancer.
Note. From The American Urological Association (2000).

Unfortunately, TRUS has limitations for use as a primary screening tool. Costs for TRUS range from $50 to $250 without a biopsy and from $200 to $800 with biopsy (Littrup, Lee, & Mettlin, 1992). Additionally, Waldman and Osborne (1994) concluded that TRUS detects only about 10% to 20% of lesions in the transitional zone of the prostate gland, has low predictive values in lesions less than 1 cm, and is operator-dependent. TRUS is not widely promoted as a primary screening test, but it is used to investigate abnormalities on the DRE and PSA measurements and to guide biopsies (Vetrosky & White, 1998).

SCREENING

Screening is the use of a test or examination to detect a disease at the early stage and to reduce disease-related mortality (Waldman & Osborne, 1994). Screening for prostate cancer involves the use of a digital rectal examination (DRE), a serum prostate-specific antigen (PSA) test, and, if appropriate, a transrectal ultrasound (TRUS). However, there is controversy among health organizations about the use of the DRE and PSA tests in asymptomatic men for routine screening methods of prostate cancer. The ACS and the American Urological Association (AUA) recommend that asymptomatic men over age 50 with at least a 10-year life expectancy should be screened annually for prostate cancer by both the DRE and the PSA tests. For men at high risk, such as those with a strong family history of prostate cancer or African American men, it may be appropriate to undergo screening at a younger age (von Eschenbach, Ho, Murphy, Cunningham, & Lins, 1997). Conversely, some health organizations, such as the National Cancer Institute (NCI) and the U.S. Preventive Services Task Force, do not endorse routine screening for prostate cancer (Gerard & Frank-Stromborg, 1998).

Arguments in favor of prostate cancer screening are based upon the belief that screening, using both the DRE and PSA, increases the detection of organ-confined prostate cancer. If prostate cancer is confined to the prostate, effective treatment is more likely, and the death rates can ultimately be reduced (Gerard & Frank-Stromborg, 1998).

Those that argue against prostate cancer screening claim that there is a lack of well-designed randomized controlled studies showing that early detection of prostate cancer, in an asymptomatic phase, significantly improves survival and reduces mortality (Coley, Barry, Fleming, Fahs, & Mulley, 1997). Furthermore, the side-effects resulting from treating prostate cancers identified as a result of early screening, such as impotence and incontinence, may be worse than the disease itself, since patients with the early disease are usually asymptomatic (Garnick, 1993). In addition, screening for the disease may be financially costly without proving that screening reduces prostate cancer mortality. It is predicted that the screening would cost the United States $12 to $28 billion (U.S. Preventive Services Task Force, 1996). Lubke, Optenberg, and Thompson (1994) estimated that the overall cost of initiating a nationwide prostate cancer screening and treatment program for all eligible men would range from $8.5 to $25.7 billion per year.

This controversy will continue until definitive answers can support that screening and aggressive treatment for prostate cancer can lower mortality rates. Two randomized, controlled trials are currently under way. They include a European randomized study of screening for prostate cancer (Schroder, 1994) and the prostate, lung, and colorectal and ovarian cancer screening trial of the National Cancer Institute (Gohagan, Prorok, Kremer, & Cornett, 1994). Results of these trials are expected around the year 2008.

Facilitators and Barriers of Prostate Cancer Screening

Even though controversy surrounds screening for early detection of prostate cancer, most clinicians and researchers agree that at-risk men, especially African American men and men with a family history of prostate cancer, need to be screened (Gelfand, Parzuchowski, Cort, & Powell, 1995; Weinrich, Weinrich, Boyd, & Atkinson, 1998). Thus, one important role of nurses may be to engage at-risk men to participate in prostate cancer screening. To do so, nurses have to consider facilitators and barriers of participation in prostate cancer screening.

Perceived benefits are significant facilitators of participation in prostate cancer screening. Based upon the Health Belief Model (Becker, 1974) and the Poverty-Cancer Model (Freeman, 1989), Tingen and her colleagues (1998) conducted a correlational study with 1,522 men. The sample included 72% African American men that were aged 40 to 70 and 28% Caucasian men aged 50 to 70 years. The purpose of the study was to examine perceived benefits as facilitators of participation in prostate cancer screening. Results indicated that men who perceived participation in prostate cancer screening as a benefit were more likely to participate in screening.

Prostate cancer knowledge has been shown to facilitate participation in screening. Weinrich, Weinrich, Boyd, and Atkinson (1998) demonstrated that men without a previous history of prostate cancer screening ($N = 319$, 82% African American) who had more knowledge of prostate cancer, were more likely to participate in a prostate cancer screening with a digital rectal examination and prostate specific antigen. Another facilitator to participation in prostate screening includes cues. McKee

(1994) noted that appointment scheduling, reminder cards prior to screening, having a friend/family member with cancer, and advertisement of screening programs in newspaper promotions would positively influence the participation in screening for prostate cancer.

Reported barriers to prostate cancer screening also include negative feelings about the DRE (Underwood, 1991). In a study of 1,395 African American men, Shelton, Weinrich, and Reynolds (1999) reported that embarrassment was a significant barrier to prostate cancer screening. Fear of cancer has been also reported as a barrier to willingness to undergo the DRE (Gelfand, Parzuchowski, Cort, & Powell, 1995). However, there are conflicting results on concern about sexual difficulties following surgery, as a barrier. Weinrich, Reynolds, Tingen, and Starr (2000) reported that inability to have sex after prostate surgery was not a barrier. Cost and lack of knowledge have been identified as barriers (Weinrich et al., 2000).

Based on the factors previously identified, nurses must educate men, especially high-risk men, on prostate cancer and its benefits and also plan strategies for cues to participation in screening. Nurses must also continue to make an effort to identify other facilitators and barriers of participation in prostate cancer screening. The existing studies mainly have explored each facilitator or barrier in a separate study. Therefore, it is difficult to understand how the facilitators and barriers together influence participation in screening for prostate cancer. Thus, it has been recommended to study the facilitators and barriers, simultaneously.

Individualized Approach for Screening

Even though mass screening for prostate cancer is controversial, the American College of Physicians has recommended that health professionals inform an individual about potential benefits and known harms of screening and let them make the decision regarding screening (Coley, Barry, & Mulley, 1997). The following information may be used with men who are considering having screening tests (Coley, Barry, & Mulley, 1997):

- Prostate cancer is an important health problem.
- The benefits of one-time or repeated screening and aggressive treatment of prostate cancer have not yet been proven.
- DRE and PSA measurement can both have false-positive and false-negative results.
- The probability that further invasive evaluation will be required as a result of testing is relatively high.

Assessment, Screening, Diagnosis 43

TABLE 3.3 Facilitators of and Barriers to the Participation in Prostate Cancer Screening

Facilitators	Barriers
• Perceived benefit	• Negative feelings (e.g., embarrassment, fear)
• Knowledge	• Lack of knowledge
• Cues to action (e.g., appointment scheduling, reminder cards)	• Cost

- Aggressive therapy is necessary to realize any benefit from the discovery of a tumor.
- A small but finite risk for early death and a significant risk for chronic illness, particularly with regard to sexual and urinary function, are associated with these treatments.
- Early treatment may save lives.
- Early detection and treatment may avert future cancer-related illness.

Volk and colleagues (1997) found that the decision for prostate cancer screening often involves spousal opinion. In an exploratory study of 10 couples, 7 of 10 husbands preferred the screening, while 9 of 10 wives preferred that their husbands undergo screening. The investigators of the study recommended that guidelines for prostate cancer screening should consider assessing the couple's preference.

DIAGNOSIS

Diagnostic Testing

If certain symptoms or the results of screening tests indicate the possibility of prostate cancer, a biopsy is commonly performed to make a definitive diagnosis. Subsequently, magnetic resonance imaging, computed tomography scans, and bone scans may also be done to detect distant metastases. Diagnostic laboratory tests commonly performed include: serum acid phosphatase, alkaline phosphatase, and calcium.

A transrectal biopsy is the most commonly used procedure for removing a small piece of tumor tissue for examination under a microscope. Biopsies are usually done under TRUS guidance so that multiple planes of the prostate anatomy can be visualized. For the tissue sampling, a spring-loaded biopsy gun with a cored needle is commonly used rather than the traditionally used Vim-Silverman or Tru-cut needles because of the advantages of less post-biopsy infection and pain (Gerber & Chodak, 1993; Hodge, McNeal, & Stamey, 1989). Usually six samples are obtained from the upper, middle, and lower areas of the left and right sides to take a representative sample of the prostate gland and identify how much of the gland is affected by the cancer. After the biopsy, hematuria and hematospermia may exist for several days to weeks. Therefore, nurses should instruct patients about these post-test side effects. Fine-needle aspiration is another form of biopsy (Snyder, 2000). Advantages of fine-needle aspiration are lower diagnostic morbidity and lower cost. However, a disadvantage of the modality is need for an experienced cytopathologist to interpret aspirated contents (Gerber & Chodak, 1993).

Computed tomography (CT) is an X-ray procedure that creates cross-sectional images of the selected body. CT of the pelvis is performed to detect pelvic lymph node enlargement; however, it may also provide valuable information regarding the size of the tumor (Montie, 2000). Magnetic resonance imaging (MRI) is used when looking for capsular penetration, pelvis lymph node metastasis, and bony metastasis. Limitations of MRI are expense and inconvenience for patients (Montie, 2000).

Radionuclide bone scan is used to detect the spread of cancer to the bones. However, bone scans may reveal false-positive images at the sites of arthritis or trauma (Carter & Partin, 1998). Bone scans are generally not necessary in men who have a PSA less than 10.0 ng/ml and no skeleton symptoms (Oesterling, Martin, Bergstralh, & Lowe, 1993).

In laboratory tests, alkaline phosphatase and calcium may be elevated in the presence of bone metastases. Serum acid phosphatase may be elevated with disease outside the confines of the prostate (Mahon, Casporson, & Wozeniak-Potrofsky, 1990).

Grading and Staging

Prostate cancer is histologically classified into grades according to the degree of differentiation found in the malignant cells at the time of biopsy. The most commonly used grading system for prostate cancer is the Gleason system. In this system, the two most common malignant cell patterns are each graded on a scale of 1 to 5. Subscores are added to indicate the total Gleason score. Gleason scores of 2 to 4 refer to well-differentiated tumors which are likely to be slow growing. Gleason scores of 5 to 6 refer to moderately differentiated tumors. Gleason scores of 8 to 10 are interpreted as poorly differentiated tumors. These tumors are likely to be aggressive and grow rapidly (Gleason & Mellinger, 1974; Vetrosky & White, Jr., 1998).

In addition to the Gleason system, prostate cancer is also staged to define the extent of cancer and to guide appropriate therapy (Montie, 2000). The most commonly used system for staging prostate cancer is the TNM staging system (Beahrs, Henson, Hutter, & Kennedy, 1992; International Union Against Cancer, 1992) (see chapter 1). In this system, T refers to the primary tumor; N refers to the level of regional nodal involvement; and M refers to the presence of distance metastases.

CONCLUSION

Nurses play a pivotal role in assessment, screening, and diagnosis of prostate cancer. Nurses assess men's risk factors for prostate cancer (e.g., age, family history, race, lifestyle, and occupational characteristics) as well as urinary signs and symptoms that may be associated with prostate cancer. Based upon the assessment, nurses may guide men at high risk toward screening for prostate cancer.

Since mass screening for prostate cancer is currently controversial, nurses must inform men at high risk of the potential benefits versus the harm of screening and then individualize the decision to screen. When discussing screening with men, nurses must consider facilitators of, and barriers to, the participation in prostate cancer screening.

Nurses educate patients about why and how the diagnostic tests are performed and help patients and their families understand the meaning of prostate cancer staging. Such nursing interventions may reduce patients' diagnosis-related stress by helping them to become knowledgeable about diagnostic tests and staging of prostate cancer.

4

Treatment Choices and the Decision-Making Process

Maureen E. O'Rourke

First a man must decide what he will not do, only then can he decide what he ought to do.

—Meniscus

Each year more than 100,000 men in the United States will be diagnosed with prostate cancer and faced with a significant life-changing decision: how to treat their disease. Decisions regarding prostate cancer treatment selection are complex. In contrast to other disease entities, where there is known best evidence and standards of practice to guide treatment decisions, prostate cancer serves as a model of scientific and personal uncertainty. Both prostate cancer screening and the choice of optimal treatment are affected by this uncertainty. Patients look to health care providers for assistance with treatment decisions, but they also look to other equally powerful information sources such as family and friends. Patients and their families bring their personal histories to the decision-making table. As they consider each option, they process this information through the filters of their own life experiences, biases about cancer and cancer treatment, the cancer experiences of others they have known, what they hear, see, and read, and advice they receive—solicited or not.

The purpose of this chapter is to outline the factors involved in decision making regarding treatment selection for early stage prostate cancer. This review will examine the available treatment options and data related to associated side effects and how consideration of these influence the ultimate treatment choice. Additionally, patient preferences, the influence of age and other contextual variables will be examined. The existence of treatment biases and the issue of who ultimately makes the treatment decision will be discussed. Finally, the literature on nursing interventions, although scant, will be reviewed.

FACTORS AFFECTING THE PROSTATE CANCER TREATMENT DECISION

Medical Models

The issue of deciding on the most appropriate prostate cancer treatment is presented in the medical literature as a collaborative process. Physicians are seen as information providers who guide patients to the optimal choice both medically and personally. Physicians themselves may rely on formal decision analysis trees to guide their own decision making. These decision trees are based on Bayesian models of statistical probability. The development of nomograms, or devices to guide individual patient outcome predications, are, in turn, based on the accumulation and integration of multiple test results and specific patient outcome predictions. Several nomograms have been developed to assist physicians in their decision making regarding the treatment of patients with clinically localized prostate cancer, including specific practice guidelines developed by the National Comprehensive Cancer Network (NCCN, 1997).

Available Treatment Options

Currently there is no consensus within the scientific community regarding optimal treatment for early stage prostate cancer. Within the confines of Western medicine, three basic options are offered: radical prostatectomy, radiation therapy (external beam or brachytherapy approach), or "Expectant Management," also referred to as "Watchful Waiting." Other treatments do exist, such as cryotherapy, and still others remain investigational (genetic therapy).

The key factors common to models designed for physician use include the patient's age, projected survival, coexisting medical conditions, stage of disease, and tumor factors such as grade and Gleason score. Additionally, consideration is given to the expected side effects associated with each treatment modality and patients' personal preferences.

Treatment options can be summarized as follows (Tester & Brouch, 2000):

- Stage I Disease: Available options include watchful waiting or careful observation without further treatment, versus more definitive treatment such as prostatectomy for younger males in otherwise good health.
- Stage II Disease: Options include radical prostatectomy, external beam radiotherapy (XRT), brachytherapy, and watchful waiting.
- Stage III Disease: Options include XRT with or without hormonal

manipulation, hormonal manipulation alone, and radical prostatectomy. Watchful waiting is an option for older men and those men who are asymptomatic but have other comorbid conditions that may limit their lifespan.

Medical Considerations Influencing the Treatment Decision

Prostate cancer is associated with the aging process. More than 75% of all cases are diagnosed among men over age 65. After age 50, both incidence and mortality rates increase nearly exponentially. Diagnosis before age 50 is associated with decreased relative survival (Brawley, Knopf, & Thompson, 1999). Histologic tumors have been documented in 70% to 90% of men over the age of 80 at autopsy (Sakr et al., 1993), leading to the conclusion that older patients may die with the disease rather than of the disease. In general, patients with a limited life expectancy are not considered candidates for radical treatment such as prostatectomy, which may incur significant morbidity.

The presence of coexisting medical conditions influences the risk of treatment-related side effects. Patients with cardiovascular, renal, and pulmonary disease are usually identified as poor surgical candidates. The incidence of these conditions rises with age, thus these factors are intimately related in the decision-making process.

Patient survival is directly related to the extent of tumor involvement. Confinement of the tumor to the prostate gland itself, without capsular penetration, is associated with survival in excess of five years. Pelvic node or seminal vesicle involvement is associated with a worse prognosis. Tumors that have spread to distant organs are considered incurable and are associated with survival of less than three years. These patients are more likely to die "of prostate cancer," than with it (Griffin & O'Rourke, 1999).

The consensus within the health care community is that for most men with early stage disease, multiple treatment options exist. The ultimate selection of treatment modality should be based on the efficacy of the treatment balanced by consideration of the potential complications that may be experienced, and the patient's views regarding quality of life. Critical to the decision is the availability of comprehensive, accurate and credible information.

Patient Preferences in Decision Making

The health care literature highlights the conflicting state of knowledge regarding the degree to which patients desire to participate in the treatment decision-making process (Blanchard, Labreque, Ruckdeschel, &

Blanchard, 1988; Cassileth, Zupkis, Sutton-Smith, & March, 1980; Degner & Sloan, 1992; Degner & Russell, 1988; O'Rourke, 1997). Interpretation across studies regarding decision-making preferences has been complicated by sampling concerns, measurement inconsistencies, and the use of hypothetical scenarios.

Davison, Degner, and Morgan (1995) examined the decision-making preferences of 57 men with prostate cancer. The majority of men sampled preferred a passive role (as defined by the researchers) in decision making. Twenty-three percent preferred a collaborative role, and 19% preferred an active role, although a large proportion of men reported that they wanted more information than they had received. The categories of "active," "passive," and "collaborative" roles were based on the researchers' definitions and may be culturally bound terms. Deferral of the treatment decision, while defined by the researchers as "passive," may have constituted an "active" decision by the men. Such a deferral may not be viewed as passive by some cultural groups, and decisional deferral to the respected authority might be viewed by some as an appropriate response. The researchers did not examine the reasons for decisional deferral to physicians, but such a choice may have resulted from a perception of inadequate information to make the decision, or an attempt to attenuate any potential blame and minimize regret if the ultimate outcome is not as desired. These researchers did not explore the role of family members in the treatment decision making process.

Other studies by Degner and Sloan (1992) have yielded similar findings, with 59% of newly diagnosed cancer patients wanting physicians to make treatment decisions on their behalf. The findings revealed that when healthy adults were faced with a hypothetical cancer diagnosis, 64% of these desired to select their own treatment.

With regard to prostate cancer specifically, one of the earliest reported investigations of prostate cancer treatment decision making was conducted by Cassileth and associates (1989). Among a convenience sample of 147 prostate cancer patients with advanced disease, 78% of men chose hormonal therapy, and 70% of these reported discussing the decision with their wives. Twenty-two percent of men chose orchiectomy, yet only 59% reported discussing this with their wives.

More recently, Mazur and Merz (1995) examined the decision-making preferences of 163 men (aged 35–84) regarding prostate cancer treatment selection. The men were presented with a hypothetical scenario of prostate cancer and were each offered a choice between two procedures, radical prostatectomy or radiation therapy. The men were shown survival curves in graph form for each treatment option (labeled options A and B to prevent bias). Treatment A (surgery) was depicted as having worse short-term side effects, but better long-term survival. Treatment B (radiation therapy) was shown to have fewer short-term side effects, but worse long-term survival. Ninety-four percent of men chose option A, favoring survival despite the high probability of incontinence and impotence. Fully 83% were willing to accept a 100% chance of impotence, while only 62% of men were willing to accept a 100% chance of incontinence, suggesting that the latter may be a more bothersome side effect exerting more influence on the treatment decision process. Despite the importance of these findings, interpretation must include consideration of the methodological flaws and limitations of this study. The age range was far too wide, and it is likely that 35-year-old men view impotence and incontinence in a different manner than their older counterparts. The differential casting of 5-year survival curves by the investigators suggesting better 5-year survival with surgery versus radiotherapy is problematic and not based on current scientific evidence. The question remains, if these men were accurately apprised of the uncertainties upon which these survival projections were based, would their decisions have been different (Fowler, 1995).

Decision-Making Preferences and Age

There is some evidence that decisional preferences change with age. Research suggests that the current older cohort, while not a homogenous group, may desire less participation in the decision process (Beisecker, 1988; Degner & Russel, 1988; Pierce, 1993). The involvement of intimate others may be a salient factor in treatment decisions by older adults. Numerous researchers have identified the tendency of older patients to be accompanied to their appointments, and this third party in the decision-making process is one of the distinguishing characteristics of the doctor-geriatric patient relationship (Greene, Majewrovitz, Adelman, & Rizzo, 1986; Coe & Prendergast, 1985). Adelman, Greene, and Charon (1987) proposed that this third person may take on the role of patient advocate, passive participant, or agonist.

The doctor-patient relationship is another factor, interacting with age, which affects decision-making preferences and styles. The changing nature of this relationship from one based on paternalism to one based on consumerism may result in role confusion for older patients who prefer, or are accustomed to, the more paternalistic mode. Older patients may also be more vulnerable to the asymmetric imbalance of power due to their cohort status (immigrant status, educational background, language barriers, socio-economic status, etc.) (O'Rourke, 1997).

Age may not only influence the patient's interpretation of the available treatment options and their personal meanings, but may be a factor affecting the information and treatment options that they receive. Some researchers have suggested that health care providers themselves are influenced by ageist beliefs, with younger patients being more likely to be referred to cancer centers where they may be offered more aggressive therapies (Burklow, 1992; Derby, 1991; MacCormick & Mackinnon, 1990).

Contextual Factors Influencing Cancer Treatment Decisions

The diagnosis of cancer and the meaning of cancer therapy are inextricably embedded in a person's global life, including their family history, personal history, personality traits, social integration, and spirituality (Haberman, 1995). Fears regarding cancer and perceptions of lack of control may influence beliefs about cancer and cancer treatments. O'Rourke (1997, 1999) observed that both patients and their spouses held deep biases against specific prostate cancer treatments such as watchful waiting and radiation therapy, and these biases precluded full consideration of these treatment options.

Although a substantial body of work exists examining racial, cultural, and ethnic influences on participation in cancer screening and prevention activities, data are just beginning to emerge regarding the influence of cultural factors on cancer treatment decisions. Cancer fatalism has been identified as one critical variable affecting differential participation in prevention activities by African Americans (Powe, 1996). Income and education have also been noted to be strong predictors. The influence of these factors on the decision-making process has not yet been fully explored.

The influence of social factors (marital status, family living at home, and parenthood status) upon treatment preferences was examined by Yellen and Cella (1995). They reported that the strongest and most consistent predictor of treatment preference was parenthood status. Parents were more likely to accept aggressive treatment associated with severe toxicity and low quality of life. Gender and marital status were not predictive of treatment preferences. Social context appears to be an important factor for consideration during the treatment-decision process.

Consideration of Treatment Side Effects

Documentation of the potential and actual side effects experienced by men following treatment for early-stage prostate cancer can be found in both the medical and lay literature. The magnitude and frequency of these side effects is difficult to ascertain, however, largely due to two factors. Consideration of the three main side effects, urinary incontinence (UI), impotence, and altered bowel functioning, has been undervalued in favor of a primary philosophical approach focusing on tumor control at all costs. Additionally, many studies have used retrospective approaches to survey the incidence, severity, and degree of bother associated with these treatment-related side effects. In reviewing the literature there is a striking disparity not only in the statistics cited, but also in the measures utilized. As the philosophical approach to cancer care has gradually shifted, there has been a growing realization that quality of life and quantity of life are not mutually exclusive. A new dimension of data has recently been included in research examining treatment-related side effects, the degree of bother men attribute to these side effects.

TREATMENT-RELATED IMPOTENCE

Interpretation of data regarding the incidence and severity of impotence is hampered by the lack of a standardized definition of impotence and by reliance on self-reports of potency levels by affected men. Although Lim and colleagues (1995) reported higher rates of impotence associated with radical prostatectomy as compared to radiation therapy, Walsh has consistently reported lower rates of impotence following radical prostatectomy utilizing a nerve-sparing technique (Walsh & Donker, 1982; Walsh, Partin, & Epstein, 1994; Walsh, Marschke, & Ricker, 2000). Walsh's most recent report cites potency rates at 3, 6, 12, and 18 months following radical prostatectomy to be 38%, 54%, 73%, and 86%, respectively (2000). Among men ages 30 to 39 at 12 to 18 months postradical prostatectomy, sexual dysfunction was reported to cause "no bother." Men aged 50 to 59 reported the highest levels of degree of bother. Recovery of potency by 18 months was correlated with age at time of surgery: 30 to 39 years, 100%; 40 to 49 years, 88%; 50 to 59 years, 90%; and 60 to 67 years, 75%.

Krupski and colleagues (2000) report similar findings related to a low degree of bother caused by sexual dysfunction among men treated with radical prostatectomy, yet conflicting results have been reported by Davis and colleagues (2000). This research team reported both higher degree of sexual functioning and lower degree of bother among men treated with brachytherapy as compared to a similar group treated with radical prostatectomy.

Watchful waiting involves no actual treatment delivery and thus is not directly linked with impotence. Sexual dysfunction may be present at diagnosis, however, or develop with disease progression. If hormonal therapy is initiated, patients will experience impotence.

TREATMENT-RELATED BOWEL DYSFUNCTION

Numerous researchers have documented bowel dysfunction associated with both XRT and brachytherapy (Davis, Kuban, Lynch, & Schellhammer, 2000; Joly et al., 1998; Yarbro & Ferrans, 1993). Bowel problems have included rectal bleeding, proctitis, diarrhea, and rectal pain. High correlations between bowel dysfunction (diarrhea) and overall quality of life have been reported (Krupski, Petroni, Bissonette, & Theodorescu, 2000). Incidence of diarrhea was much higher among men treated with brachytherapy combined with XRT versus men treated with brachytherapy alone or radical prostatectomy in at least this same study (Krupski et al., 2000). When comparing bowel dysfunction among men treated with XRT versus brachytherapy, Davis and colleagues (2000) found no significant differences in either function or degree of bother. Bowel dysfunction has generally not been found to be significantly correlated with radical prostatectomy. However, bowel dysfunction is associated with XRT and brachytherapy, and these treatments may accompany surgical treatment. Bowel dysfunction is not associated with the "watch and wait" approach to early stage prostate cancer.

TREATMENT-RELATED URINARY INCONTINENCE

The incidence of postoperative urinary incontinence (UI) following radical prostatectomy ranges from 3% to 69% (Bates, Wright, & Gillatt, 1998; Fenely, Gillat, Hehir, & Kirby, 1996). Cespedes and colleagues (1999), however, report a range varying from 2% to 87% in their review. Low estimates may be reflective of samples including larger numbers of younger men. Griffiths and Neal (1997) reported that patients older than 70 years had double the incontinence rates of younger cohorts.

In the immediate postoperative period, UI has been reported to be nearly universal. Recovery is generally seen within 2 to 12 months (Cespedes et al., 1999). Research by Talcott and associates (1998) draws attention to the lingering nature of UI. This team reported that 58% of radical prostatectomy patients continued to use absorbent pads at 3 months post surgery, and 35% continued to use pads at 12 months post radical prostatectomy. Additionally, within this sample 5% of men treated with radical prostatectomy were using penile clamps to control incontinence.

In a prospective study, Davidson and colleagues (1996) followed 180 men treated with radical prostatectomy. Immediately following catheter removal, UI requiring the use of absorbent pads was reported by 56% of respondents. The initial mean measured urinary loss was 226 ml per

24 hour period, although the volume was not predictive of time to continence recovery. At three months postsurgery, 21% remained incontinent. Fourteen percent of men continued to require absorbent pads at 12 months. Eleven men received artificial sphincters and recovered continence.

Higher rates of UI have been reported among men treated with radical prostatectomy as compared to radiation therapy (Lim, Brandon, Fiedler, Brickman, Boyer, Raub, et al., 1995). Fowler and colleagues (1996) reported that a significantly higher number of post prostatectomy patients used pads or penile clamps as compared to only 7% among the radiation group). In contrast, the Johns Hopkins group reported that in their series ($n = 64$) 93% of men self-reported continence (requiring no pad usage) and 98% self-reported no or small bother related to UI at 12 months postradical prostatectomy (Walsh, Marschke, Ricker, & Burnett, 2000).

Perhaps even more important, Lim's research team documented that UI had a significant positive association with tension, fatigue, and depression (1995). A significant negative association was noted between UI and a sense of vigor and social well-being among men in their study. An inverse relationship between UI and time interval after surgery was also noted, indicating that UI may diminish over time, even without intervention. Although UI may lessen over time, quality of life is significantly affected by UI.

Age has been examined as a factor influencing post prostatectomy UI. Men under age 65 reported less UI at both 3 and 12 months postradical prostatectomy as compared with similarly treated men who were over age 65 (Talcott et al., 1998), and this difference could not be explained by presurgery status. Catalona and colleagues (1999) also found an association between age and UI recovery rates, but failed to document any association with other factors such as tumor volume, stage, or type of surgery (nerve sparing or non-nerve sparing).

UI is also a significant side effect of external beam radiation therapy (XRT). Interpretation of incidence rates is complicated by a lack of consistency in measurement intervals, definitions of UI, and the fact that radiation therapy is often coupled with other treatment modalities. Griffiths and Neal (1997) reported the overall incidence of UI following XRT as 3% to 7%. Lee and colleagues (1996) studied 758 patients and reported that only four patients experienced UI necessitating the use of one or less incontinence pads per day. The reported actuarial rate of incontinence at 5 years post-RT was 1% to 3%. Men who had a history of prior transurethral prostate resection (TURP) had significantly higher rates than those who had TURP alone.

Despite the consistent data suggesting that XRT-related incontinence is significantly less than radical prostatectomy-related incontinence (Potosky et al., 2000; Yarbro & Ferrans, 1998), at least one study has identified men in the XRT treatment group as perceiving UI to be worse than men in the surgery group. Perception of degree of bother associated with UI may be more important to men than the actual degree of incontinence itself.

Brachytherapy is becoming an increasingly popular treatment option for men with early stage prostate cancer. Freedom from relapse (as defined by biochemical markers—prostate specific antigen [PSA]) is reportedly similar to that achieved following radical prostatectomy (Blasko, Wallner, Grimm, & Ragde, 1995; Wallner, Lee, Wasserman, & Dattoli, 1997). Although the incidence appears to be low, UI is associated with brachytherapy. In a sample treated with brachytherapy, urinary symptoms including hesitancy, nocturia, frequency, and dysuria were most pronounced within the first few months after treatment, with gradual lessening over time. In another study, the prevalence of dysuria 6 months posttreatment was 10%, hesitancy 25%, nocturia 15%, and 35% for diminished force of urinary stream, a risk factor for the development of urinary retention (Arterbery, Frazier, Dalmia, Siefer, Lutz, & Porter, 1997). Wallner and associates (1997) reported low incidence of UI among men undergoing prostatic implants of iodine 125, even among men who were previously treated with TURPs. These data should be interpreted with caution when compared to other studies (Blasko et al., 1995), suggesting higher rates of UI among men previously treated with TURPs. The results from Wallner's study may differ because a 2-month waiting period prior to brachytherapy was required of men who had undergone TURPS. This delay may have led to improved outcomes by allowing time for urethral healing. Among Wallner's group, only 1 of 19 men developed mild stress UI at 6 months postimplantation. Actuarial estimates drawn from this study suggest a 6% risk of UI among these same men at 3 years posttreatment (1997).

Comparisons of quality of life and treatment side effects among men treated with brachytherapy alone, brachytherapy in combination with XRT, and radical prostatectomy suggest that men receiving combination therapy with implants and XRT have significantly lower overall quality of life when compared to the other treatment groups (Krupski, Petroni, Bissonette, & Theodorescue, 2000). In this study, the men treated with radical prostatectomy reported fewer irritative and obstructive urinary symptoms. The brachytherapy alone group had more urinary symptoms at six months when compared to the radical prostatectomy group. Both the brachytherapy and combined brachytherapy and XRT groups did show improvement over time (Krupski et al., 2000). Early reports suggest conflicting findings regarding the association between UI and brachytherapy, although some tendency toward low UI incidence has been reported.

Cryotherapy represents a new treatment option for prostate cancer. This treatment involves the direct application of ice to the prostate gland via percutaneously inserted cryogenic probes. Reported complications include UI, urethral sloughing, and bladder neck contracture. Wong's research team (1997) reported using the new techniques which include continuous temperature monitoring to treat 83 men with stage II disease (84%) or stage II disease and higher (16%). Some men had received prior surgery or XRT. Treatment success rates were impressive, with 90% of men having negative follow-up biopsies. PSA levels dropped from a mean of 11.2 to 0.3 at 30 months posttreatment. Despite these encouraging findings, complication rates were high: 47% of men experienced urethral sloughing as a result of prostatic urethral necrosis. Forty-four percent of these men required TURPs. Among men who had received prior radiation therapy, 57% experienced severe incontinence. Men treated with prior surgery had higher incontinence rates than others in the study. Men with no prior treatment experienced the least UI, at the rate of 4%.

Cryotherapy may have potential as an alternative treatment form for prostate cancer, however, its long-term efficacy compared with more well-established treatment modalities has yet to be determined. Early studies indicate significant urinary side effects, some of which require surgical intervention for correction (Wong, Chinn, Chinn, & Tom, 1997). Further investigation is needed to determine its efficacy and the incidence, severity, duration, and degree of bother caused by treatment related UI.

Side Effects and Treatment Choices

Given the present state of the knowledge, it is understandable that if health care providers remain uncertain about both the incidence of treatment-related impotence, incontinence, and bowel dysfunction and the degree of bother each causes, patients and their families may not be able to process this information and its personal meaning to assist them in reaching a treatment decision. How treatment side effect information is presented by health care providers and how this information is interpreted by patients and their partners affects their ultimate treatment choice.

Some research has been conducted examining treatment preferences of men and their spouses regarding the trade-off of symptoms for survival gains. Mazur and Merz (1995) suggested that men may be willing to accept a high risk of side effects in return for enhanced longevity. In one study (Volk, Cantor, Spann, Cass, Cardenas, & Warren, 1997), women were more likely than men to opt for more radical treatment choices than their spouses when presented with hypothetical prostate cancer scenarios. Women were motivated by a desire to prolong time together with their husbands. Conversely, men were more conservative with regard to treatment choices, and rated impotence and incontinence as more burdensome side effects than did their wives. Men even stated that they might be inclined to forego some treatment options due to their potential side effects (Volk et al., 1997). O'Rourke's research corroborated this finding (1997). In her study involving 18 couples, both patients and their spouses expressed concern over potential treatment-related side effects; however, women, when interviewed privately, stated that their marital longevity would lessen their worry about the effects of impotence and incontinence on their marital relationship. The women emphasized their desire to prolong time together as a couple. In their own private interviews men did not identify marital longevity as an attenuating factor. Instead, some men discussed the possibility of rejecting surgery because of concern over impotence and incontinence.

O'Rourke (1997) further explored sources of information related to treatment side effects. She noted that while physicians were identified as being a major information source regarding treatment-related side effects, study participants also identified friends, neighbors, and other family members who had experienced cancer. The stories they told regarding vicarious cancer experiences suggested that these were powerful influences on their treatment decision. Several couples incorrectly identified the risk of impotence and incontinence to be much higher with radiotherapy, despite being given information by their physicians to the contrary. At times they were unable to recall information about side effects, and even attributed incorrect information to their physicians. These findings suggest that although our informed consent system is predicated on factual information, discerning what pre-existing knowledge of cancer and cancer treatment families have and exploring its underlying personal meaning is critical to assisting them to select the appropriate individualized treatment.

Treatment-Related Biases

Biases related to specific cancer treatments have been underexplored in the health care literature. Data from O'Rourke's studies (1997, 1999; O'Rourke & Germino, 1998) suggest that underlying biases in favor of surgery and against radiotherapy deserve further investigation. She reported that couples dismissed the watch and wait option almost immediately and demonstrated a distinct bias favoring surgery as the treatment of choice. Watch and wait was described by men and their wives as "doing nothing," and was associated with painful and certain death. Participants in O'Rourke's studies also noted the influence of the media. The much publicized diagnoses of former Senator Robert Dole and General Norman Schwarzkopf were mentioned by men and their wives. The "take charge" attitude of the general may have been particularly meaningful to the men in this study, many of whom were of the World War II cohort.

O'Rourke (1997, 1999) also described the attitudes of men and their wives toward surgery and radiotherapy. Surgery was identified as the only treatment that was curative. Radiotherapy was viewed as a treatment used to slow the spread of cancer but not as a treatment that could totally eradicate the disease. Radiation was discussed as causing severe skin burns and carried with it the negative association that it is a cause of cancer, making it illogical as a treatment modality. Unfortunately few patients in O'Rourke's studies met with radiation oncologists to discuss this treatment option, thus their misconceptions remained unchallenged. Treatments were systematically ruled out based on what men were not willing to endure. In some cases, however, surgical treatment was selected immediately, even before other options were discussed. These data suggest that treatment-related biases require exploration by nurses and physicians prior to any substantive discussion of treatment options.

Who Makes the Decision?

The principle of autonomy dictates that patients have the right to make their own health decisions. Recent literature, however, has suggested that many health care decisions are not made by the patients themselves, or even the patients in concert with their physician. With regard to prostate cancer specifically, wives have been found to be intimately involved in the screening decision process (Volk et al., 1997), and in the treatment-decision making process as well (O'Rourke, 1997; O'Rourke & Germino, 1998, 1999). The significance of the spouse in treatment decisions has also been noted in the breast cancer literature (Degner & Sloan, 1992; Valanis & Rumpler, 1982; Ward, Heidrich, & Wolberg, 1989). Although breast and prostate cancer treatment differ in that there is an established body of scientific evidence documenting the equi-effectiveness of lumpectomy, coupled with radiotherapy and modified radical mastectomy, the findings from these studies may parallel some of those experienced by men with prostate cancer in that both diseases affect sexuality and body image. Both malignancies also threaten gender identity and perceptions of femininity or masculinity, and pose a threat to the marital relationship.

Three family roles in medical decision making have been described by Reust and Mattingly (1996). These are identified as: being affected by the decision, supporting, and advocating for patient autonomy. Spouses in O'Rourke's study (1997; O'Rourke & Germino, 1998) publically identified their roles as consistent with those cited by Reust and Mattingly (1996). They spoke of how the diagnosis and treatment would affect their lives and their interest in extending their couple time together. Additionally the spouses spoke of and demonstrated emotional support to their affected partners, and advocated for their autonomy. They identified that the decision belonged to their husbands, as they were the ones who must undergo the treatment and whose bodies were affected. In private interviews, however, the women described their role as much more active with some revealing that this decision would be their responsibility as were most other important family decisions. Wives in O'Rourke's studies (O'Rourke, 1997; O'Rourke & Germino, 1998) took on additional roles such as that of the record keeper. During interviews they were able to cite specific data including dates, lab values, and so forth. This role was also identified by Heyman and Rosner (1996). Wives identified themselves as educators and motivators as well.

Implicit marital decision-making styles have been described by Sillars and Kalblesch (1989) as decisions that are reached through implied and silent agreement, occurring in a conscious or unconscious manner. Both the men and their wives in O'Rourke's study (1997) spoke of intuitively "knowing" what the other spouse would think or choose.

Nursing Interventions

A goal of health care providers within the North American culture has been to enhance patient participation in their own health care decisions. Recent research efforts have focused on assisting men to take a more active role in the prostate cancer treatment decision process. The type of information that men cite as being needed as they work toward a treatment decision includes information on the course of the disease, treatment options, and disease progression (Feldman et al., 2000). Additionally, the need to discuss past cancer experiences and the cancer experiences of friends and family members along with specific information as to how these experiences compared with their own was identified (O'Rourke, 1997; O'Rourke & Germino, 1998).

Efforts to categorize the informational needs and preferences of prostate cancer patients resulting in a streamlined core of information that should be presented to all patients facing a prostate cancer treatment decision have been unsuccessful. Feldman-Stewart and colleagues (2000) surveyed 56 early-stage prostate cancer patients in their efforts to ascertain what information they considered essential in making their treatment decision. Given a list of 93 questions, men were asked to rank them as essential/desired, or nonessential/avoid. No single question emerged as being relevant to more than 50% of the participants. Ninety-one of the 93 questions were considered essential/desired to at least one patient. The researchers concluded that no core set of essential questions could be developed and that information needs are highly subjective and thus counseling should be highly individualized.

Several studies have focused on interventions to enhance decision making. Davison and Degner (1997) examined the effects of a self-efficacy intervention on participation in the treatment decision process, and on anxiety. The intervention itself entailed a discussion session with a nurse with extensive experience in the area of treatment decision making. During the session a list of questions was reviewed, giving the men a starting point as to where to begin when asking questions of their doctor. Patients were also encouraged to add specific questions of their own to the list and were explicitly shown where specific information was located in the resource packet that they received. Men were also given an audiotape and encouraged to record their discussion with their physician for later referral. At 6 weeks post intervention, men in the self-efficacy group took on a significantly more active role in the decision process and had lower state anxiety levels than men in the control group who were provided with written information only.

Other researchers have used a videotaped intervention in their efforts to enhance shared decision making (Volk, Cass, & Spann, 1999). While this study focused on shared decision making with regard to PSA testing, the finding may also have implications for treatment decision making as well. Baseline knowledge regarding PSA testing was low, but at 2-week follow-up participants demonstrated a 78% improvement in the number of knowledge questions they were able to answer correctly. No significant differences were noted in the control group. Interestingly, only 62% of the intervention group indicated that they planned to have a PSA test as compared to 80% of the control group. The researchers concluded that the educational intervention resulted in more informed decision making. The finding that the control group was more likely to plan to have a PSA test suggests that information may have been delivered or was interpreted in a manner that deterred participants in the intervention group from pursuing this screening test.

A hypermedia program integrating CD-ROM and Internet technology was developed by Jenkinson and colleagues (1998) in an attempt to assist newly diagnosed prostate cancer patients with knowledge acquisition expected to enhance their decision making. Results of the pilot test ($n = 10$) suggested that users found the program to be useful, relevant, and navigable, but outcomes on decision making were not reported.

The method of communicating risk information and the outcomes of prostate cancer treatment decision making has also been explored. Mazur, Hickam, and Mazur (1999) noted that among those who preferred surgical risk information to be presented numerically, the tendency to choose "surgery now" was higher. This single study suggests that the method of communication may influence the ultimate treatment choice.

Physicians may be more optimistic in their utility assessments regarding quality of life expectations than patients themselves. Decision analytic models may allow for more explicit quantification of expected benefits, toxicities, and patient preferences. Soucheck and colleagues (2000) challenge this recommendation. In their own research they detected inconsistencies in rank ordering of health states and illogical utility assessments made by patients, leading them to conclude that such methods may have serious validity problems.

Intervention studies are just now beginning to be developed and tested in an effort to assist men as they seek information necessary to make informed prostate cancer treatment decisions, and to cope with the uncertainty associated with these decisions. Interventions have employed a variety of methods aimed at improving information access and retention. Given the available data regarding the decision-making process itself, information alone is unlikely to lessen the burden of uncertainty. Allowing patients and the family members of their choice to discuss their fears, biases, and past experiences with cancer and cancer treatment appears to be an integral component of any intervention. Interventions to deal with the lingering uncertainty in the aftermath of treatment also await development and testing.

CONCLUSION

The prostate cancer treatment selection decision is a model of complexity and uncertainty. Until sufficient data from randomized controlled studies become available to allow true comparison of both the long- and short-term outcomes of the surgical, radiotherapeutic, or watch and wait approaches, patients, their partners, and health care providers must make treatment decisions with incomplete information. Although computer-assisted analytic models may guide physicians in their counseling, research has suggested that patients and their families base their decisions on far more than factual data and actuarial predictions. Information from unlimited formal and informal resources, as well as innate personal biases, influence treatment decisions. As more becomes known about the prostate cancer treatment decision-making process, research is shifting toward the development of theory-based nursing interventions.

5
Quality of Life with Prostate Cancer

Lorrie L. Powel and Meredith Wallace

The construct of quality of life (QOL) has risen to an outcome measure of significant consequence and an important factor in the nursing care and management of many health problems. Several factors have helped to shape the direction of QOL as an endpoint of health care research in general and prostate cancer in particular: 1) consumer demand; 2) medical advances with multiple clinical choices for treatment, which leave QOL as the determinant of choice; 3) the growing number of elderly and individuals with chronic disease; 4) regulatory authorities that request QOL outcome data for drug and device approval; and 5) a trend toward more holistic care (King et al., 1997; Kinney, Burfitt, Stullenbarger, & DeBolt, 1996).

Records reporting the significance of individual QOL as a noble characteristic of health care have been chronicled in every society since Aristotle (Goodyear & Fraumeni, 1996); however, the organizing framework for contemporary definitions of QOL in patient care is derived from the World Health Organization's (WHO) definition of health: "... a state of complete physical, mental, and social well-being and not merely the absence of disease and infirmity" (WHO Chronicles, 1958, p. 11). This postwar definition symbolized a new way of thinking about the meaning of health. In so doing, it also inspired the first formal measure of QOL, the Karnofsky Scale. This measure, while highly regarded and still in use today, is unidimensional, and therefore cannot capture what we now know to be the multidimensional nature of QOL. However, both the WHO definition and this measure were important stepping stones to the instruments in use today and led to a progression of discussions which helped evolve our understanding of QOL. For example, in the 1960s discussions of QOL centered on the term *well-being*, on QOL in health care in the 1970s (Goodyear & Fraumeni, 1996). Current research focuses on health-related quality of life (HRQOL), which is a multidimensional construct that represents the burden of those experiencing disease or its treatment (Aaronson, 1988). The development and explication of the concept of QOL has progressed during the past three decades through continued QOL research and instrument development. A Medline literature search suggested over 1,100 annual entries in the past decade, illustrating the expanding scope of the concept of QOL in health care research and its important connection to the traditional outcomes of morbidity and mortality.

This chapter will explore the concept of QOL. Defining characteristics and definitions, as well as methodologic and measurement issues, will be reviewed and evaluated. QOL studies conducted with prostate cancer patients will be summarized and critiqued. The chapter will conclude with a synthesis of what is known about the concept and implications for future nursing research and practice.

Defining Characteristics

Initially questions of quality of life in clinical trials were "tacked on" to studies whose bona fide goal was survival or toxicity measurement. Research during the past 40 years has given rise to trials that focus specifically on quality of life. This has illuminated many of the difficulties inherent in measuring this subjective concept. Probably the most basic problem in measuring quality of life is defining it.

At its most fundamental level, QOL reflects one's happiness or degree of well-being (Sartorius, 1987). Two constructs appear consistently in most QOL articles: 1) individualism (Oleson, 1990), the idea that feelings, thoughts, and behaviors related to an individual's experience are unique; and 2) multidimensionality (Ferrans, 1990), the perspective that multiple aspects or dimensions make up one's experience.

Other attributes of quality of life include health and physical functioning, psychological and spiritual well-being, social roles, economic stability, and family functioning (Aaronson 1988; Ferrans, 1990; Padilla, Ferrell, Grant, & Rhiner, 1990). Another significant aspect in the assessment of quality of life is the degree of importance the individual places on the specific dimensions (Ferrans, 1990; Flanagan, 1982).

Definitions

As the measurement of QOL has evolved, researchers have used synonymous terms, including well-being, health status, functional status, and life satisfaction. Each concept presumes a slightly different meaning, which implies the use of research questions, methodologies, instruments, and methods of reporting that relate to the specific concept used. In addition, concepts may be operationalized differently among researchers. Few studies define what *they* mean by quality of life, and the overwhelming majority of studies examine one dimension of QOL—usually physical function. Similarly, few studies are based on a preexisting theoretical model or framework.

Methodologic and Measurement Issues

Ideally measurement of HRQOL should integrate indices that capture the breadth and the essence of the illness or treatment experience (Aaronson, 1988; Litwin, Hays, Ganz, Leake, & Brook, 1998; Ware, 1984). In prostate cancer research, this can be difficult because quality of life may be studied from a number of different perspectives. For example, studies may focus on quality of life in men who have experienced a certain type of treatment (e.g., surgery, radiation therapy, watchful waiting), type of surgery (e.g., nerve sparing or non-nerve sparing), symptoms (e.g., urinary incontinence, bowel or erectile dysfunction) or disease trajectory (e.g., early stage vs. metastatic disease) (Albertsen, Aaronson, Muller, Keller, & Ware, 1997; Fowler et al., 1993; Lim et al., 1995; Litwin et al., 1995; Shrader-Bogen, Kjellberg, McPherson, & Murray, 1997).

Other issues that make HRQOL measurement difficult are the subjectivity and accuracy of patient self-reports (Litwin & McGuigan, 1999) and the discrepancy between physician and patient perception of symptoms (Ojdeby, Claezon, Brekkan, Haggman, & Nolan, 1996). In studies of prostate cancer, these issues account for the wide discrepancy in outcomes reported in the literature.

To adequately assess the dimensions or attributes of health that capture the illness or treatment experience, measurement of HRQOL should ideally include indices of global QOL, disease-specific QOL, and domain- or dimension-specific QOL (Aaronson, 1988; Litwin et al., 1998; Ware, 1984). Measurement biases will be further reduced when investigators are able to conceptualize the issues to be investigated and communicate these to the respondent. Moreover, respondents must be able to read and understand the questions, recall the relevant information, and devote effort to answering the questions (Fayers & Jones, 1983).

GLOBAL QOL

Generic instruments focus on measurement of global QOL across different populations and outcomes. Examples of general HRQOL instruments used in studies of prostate cancer patients include the medical outcomes study (MOS) 36-item short form (SF-36) (Ware & Sherbourne, 1992) and the Quality of Life Index (QLI) (Ferrans & Powers, 1985). The SF-36 is self-administered multidimensional measure of HRQOL inclusive of eight constructs. It includes subscales on physical functioning, emotional well-being, health perceptions, social functioning, role limitations, pain, and energy/fatigue. It was previously developed and published by RAND researchers and is used worldwide as a measure of HRQOL. It has been used in many studies of patients with prostate cancer. (Examples of global QOL instruments are summarized in Table 5.1).

The QLI was designed to measure the satisfaction with and importance of various life domains to individual subjects. It includes items related to the following domains: health care, physical health and functioning, marriage, family, friends, stress, standard of living, occupation, education, leisure, future retirement, peace of mind, personal faith, life goals, personal appearance, self-acceptance, general happiness, and general satisfaction.

CANCER-SPECIFIC QOL

Cancer-specific instruments include items that relate to one's experience with cancer. Generally they contain items related to global QOL in the patient with cancer. These measures are not intended to be responsive to individual changes related to specific cancers or particular symptoms or syndromes. Examples include the Multidimensional Quality of Life Scale-Cancer (MQOLS-CA), the Cancer Rehabilitation Evaluation Survey Short Form (CARES), the European Organization for Research and Treatment of Cancer-Quality of Life Questionnaire-C-33 (EORTC-C-33), and the Functional Assessment of Cancer Therapy (FACT).

The MQOLS-CA is a 30-item instrument that measures four dimensions: psychosocial existential well-being, physical functional well-being, symptom distress, and worry (Padilla et al., 1996). The CARES focuses on the impact of cancer on functional status and lifestyle. It has one global rating and subscales that measure physical, psychosocial, medical interaction, marital interaction, and sexual attributes (Schag, Ganz, & Heinrich, 1991). The EORTC-C-33 is a 33-item questionnaire that incorporates five subscales related to HRQOL in patients with cancer (Aaronson et al., 1993). It has been used in studies of patients with locoregional, metastatic, and hormone resistant prostate cancer. The FACT is a 33-item general quality of life measure commonly used in oncology clinical trials for evaluating patients receiving cancer treatment (Cella et al., 1993). It includes the FACT-G (general) and various subscales developed for specific populations and treatment parameters (e.g., Fact-O for ovarian

TABLE 5.1 Examples of Global QOL Instruments

Instrument	Objective	Number of Items	Administration Mode	Time Frame
SF-36	To assess health status in patients with general medical illness	36	Interviewer, self, or proxy	Past month
NHP	To measure perceived health in patients with general medical illness	38	Self	Present
QWB	To assess health-related quality of life in patients who have received clinical therapy	18	Trained interviewer	Present
SIP	To assess QOL in patients with general medical illnesses	136	Self	Present

SF-36 = Medical Outcomes Study (MOS) 36-Item Short Form; NHP = Nottingham Health Profile; QWB = Quality of Well-being Scale; SIP = Sickness Impact Profile cancer, and Fact-T used to measure QOL in patients receiving Taxol® chemotherapy). Subscales are used in tandem with the FACT-G, allowing the capacity of both a global and a disease- or treatment-specific measure. (Examples of cancer-specific QOL instruments are summarized in Table 5.2.)

DISEASE-SPECIFIC QOL

Disease-specific instruments are designed to measure specific constructs related to the experience of patients with a particular disease (e.g., prostate cancer). For example, "Does having prostate cancer interfere with your daily activities?" Overall, these measures are insensitive to differences between groups of patients with diseases other than those they are developed to measure. Since many of the disease-specific instruments designed for prostate cancer studies measure constructs central to men with metastatic disease (e.g., hormonal changes, nausea, and vomiting), they also may not be relevant to all men with prostate cancer, such as those with early stage disease. Although disease-specific measures may include individual items that reflect symptom change, invariably they are insensitive to specific symptomatology. (Examples of disease-specific QOL instruments are summarized in Table 5.3.)

An instrument commonly used in studies of prostate cancer is the University of California at Los Angeles-Prostate Cancer Index (UCLA-PCI), developed by Litwin and colleagues (1995). It contains a total of 28 items presented in a three- to five-point Likert format. The first 11 items are from the SF-36 (Ware & Sherbourne, 1992). The remaining items relate to six subscales: urinary, bowel, and sexual function, and urinary, bowel, and sexual bother.

CONDITION-SPECIFIC QOL

There is a paucity of domain- or condition-specific instruments related to prostate cancer treatment morbidity. An item on a condition-specific instrument might be illustrated by the following example: "Do you consider the accidental loss of urine a problem that interferes with your day-to-day activities or bothers you in other ways?" (Robinson et al., 1998). Many of the instruments that measure symptoms of men after prostate cancer treatment have been developed as symptom-specific instruments for other populations (e.g., measures of urinary incontinence have been predominately focused on women) and as yet have not been well validated in men with prostate cancer.

TABLE 5.2 Examples of Cancer-Specific QOL Instruments

Instrument	Objective	Number of Items	Administration Mode	Time Frame
CARES-SF	To assess quality of life in patients with cancer	57	Self	Past month
EORTC QLQ-C30	To assess health-related quality of life in prostate cancer patients	30	Self	Past 7 days
FLIC	To measure quality of life in patients with cancer	22	Self	Present
FACT-G	To assess functional status in patients who have received cancer therapy	28	Self	Past 4 weeks
QLI-C-FP	To assess quality of life in terms of life satisfaction in patients with cancer	68	Self	Present
RSCL	To assess psychological and physical distress in patients with cancer	27	Interviewer	Past 7 days

CARES-SF = Cancer and Rehabilitation Evaluation Scales—Short form; EORTC QLQ-C30 = European Organization for Research & Treatment of Cancer Quality of Life Questionnaire, FLIC = Functional Living Index—Cancer; FACT-G = Functional Assessment of Cancer Therapy—General; QLI-C-FP = Quality of Life Index—Cancer Version; RSCL = Rotterdam Symptom Checklist

TABLE 5.3 Examples of Prostate Cancer-Specific QOL Instruments

Instrument	Objective	Number of Items	Administration Mode	Time Frame
FACT-P	To assess functional status in patients with prostate cancer	12 (47 with FACT-G)	Self	Past 7 days
UCLA-PCI	To assess health-related quality of life in prostate cancer patients	20	Self	Past month
PROSQOLI	To measure clinical outcome in men with advanced hormone-resistant prostate cancer	20	Self	Past 24 hours
PTCO-Q	To assess patients' perceptions of the incidence and severity of specific changes in bowel, urinary, and sexual function	Not reported	Self	Present

FACT-P = Functional Assessment of Cancer Therapy—Prostate Cancer; UCLA-PCI = University of California, Los Angeles Prostate Cancer Index; PROSQOLI = Prostate Cancer Specific Quality of Life Instrument; PCTO-Q = Prostate Treatment Outcomes Questionnaire.

Prostate cancer and its treatment may produce long-lasting physical sequelae that result in urinary incontinence, impotence, and bowel dysfunction. Therefore, instruments that measure both the nature and severity of symptoms, the degree of distress, and the importance to the patient are necessary.

QUALITY OF LIFE IN PROSTATE CANCER PATIENTS—A SUMMARY OF THE LITERATURE

This review focuses on select groups of studies that illustrate many of the previously mentioned difficulties inherent in studying QOL in patients with prostate cancer. Most studies in the literature have focused on physical function and therefore that is the focus of this review.

In a cross-sectional, descriptive study, Litwin and colleagues (1995) used a mail survey to determine the effect of radiation, radical prostatectomy, or watchful waiting on HRQOL. Three hundred and twenty-one men selected from a tumor registry were mailed the survey with 255 men responding (79% response rate). A population-based control group of 598 men was randomly selected from computer records of a managed care plan and matched by age and zip code. Of the control sample, 273 men responded (46% response rate). The battery of standardized instruments included a demographic questionnaire and four measures of HRQOL, the Cancer Rehabilitation Evaluation System—Short Form (CARES-SF) (Ganz, Schag, Lee, & Sim, 1992), the RAND 36-item health survey (Ware & Sherbourne, 1992), the Functional Assessment of Cancer Therapy—General Form (FACT-G) (Schipper, Clinch, McMurray, & Levitt, 1984), and an unnamed instrument that focused on the symptoms of prostate cancer (now known as the UCLA Prostate Cancer Index [UCLA-PCI], Litwin et al., 1998).

Controlling for age, analysis of covariance (ANCOVA) showed no difference in overall QOL between the three treatment groups and the comparison group. Standardized scores on each of the subscales ranged from a low score of 55.2 for the watchful waiting on the Physical Role Functioning component to a high of 81.3 for the radiation group in the Social Functioning Scale. These score reports indicate low to moderate health status across treatment groups. Significant group differences were seen between groups on sexual functioning ($F = 25.73, p < .001$) and urinary functioning ($F = 33.90; p < .001$), with the watchful waiting group experiencing the highest functioning, followed by the radiation and surgery groups. As might have been expected, men in the watchful waiting group demonstrated the best physical function, followed by radiation and surgery patients.

Significant differences were seen in role functioning ($F = 3.15; p = .02$) between each level of treatment group and the comparison group, with the radiation group demonstrating the best role function, followed by the surgery group, and the watchful waiting group. Those in the watchful waiting group also experienced the highest quality interaction with their medical provider, followed by subjects in the surgery and radiation groups.

In a study conducted by Kornblith, Herr, Ofman, Scher, and Holland (1994), survey methodology was used to determine the effect of prostate cancer treatment on the QOL of patients and spouses/partners seen in medical oncology and surgical practices. The survey included three measures (EORTC QLQ-C30 [Aaronson et al., 1993], Selby's QL Uniscale [Selby, Chapman, Etazadi-Amoli, Dalley, & Boyd, 1984], and a stress measure—Intrusion subscale of the Impact of Event Scale [Horowitz, Wilner, & Alvarez, 1979]), distributed and collected at seven lectures about prostate cancer at the Memorial Sloan-Kettering Cancer Center.

Fifty-five percent of the subjects received androgen ablation therapy for advanced disease, 28% had undergone radical prostatectomy or radiation, and 18% received no treatment for their prostate cancer. The mean age of the patients and spouse/partners was 68 and 63 years, respectively. Ninety-six percent of the patients were White, 80% were married, 48% were working, and 61% had a college degree. Thirty-six percent of spouses were employed and 41% had a college degree.

Multivariate analysis of variance (MANOVA) showed no significant difference in overall QOL among the three treatment groups on the Selby Uniscale. The investigators did not report the individual scores, but stated that all three groups experienced distress that impacted their QOL, as measured by the Intrusion Subscale of the Impact of Event Scale. Significant differences were seen in the sexual problems ($F = 15.15$, $p < .001$) and physical symptoms ($F = 6.85; p = .002$) domains of the EORTC-QLQ-C30, with the hormonal therapy group reporting the greatest difficulty, followed by the prostatectomy/radiation group. Subjects who received hormone therapy also reported the lowest QOL; this is likely due to the severe side effects of the treatment as well as their advanced stage of disease. Spouses reported significantly greater psychological distress than patients across treatment groups.

Borghede, Karlsson, and Sullivan (1997) conducted a mail survey to determine dimensions of quality of life in prostate cancer patients 1.5 to 3.5 years following diagnosis, and to test construct validity in a HRQOL instrument. Two-thousand and fifty prostate cancer patients with a mean age of 74.2 years were identified from a cancer registry in Sweden. Of the total sample, 1,138 completed surveys (55% response rate). Of these, 925 had localized prostate cancer for which 399 received watchful waiting treatment, 175 received radical prostatectomy or radiation, and 351 received palliative endocrine treatment. Subjects were asked to complete the EORTC-QLQ-C30 and an additional module was added to measure symptoms specific to patients with prostate cancer, for example, sexual, urinary, and bowel symptoms.

Factor analysis revealed three factors with eigenvalues greater than 1.0. They were the dimensions of sexual, bowel, and urinary symptoms, totaling 11 items. This underscores the importance of these three constructs as dimensions of QOL among men receiving the three treatments for prostate cancer. Only two factors with eigenvalues greater than 1.0 were extracted from the watchful waiting group. These two factors included items on sexuality (factor 1) and urinary symptoms (factor 2). Bowel factors were not extracted for this group, which lends support to the clinical absence of bowel symptoms in the watchful waiting treatment group (Held et al., 1994). Reliability (Cronbach's alpha) for the sexuality scale ranged from .68 to .90 for all treatment groups. For the urinary scale, Cronbach's alpha ranged from .50 to .73 for the three treatment groups. On the bowel factor, Cronbach's alpha ranged from .42 to .68 for the treatment groups. The investigators reported standardized scores ranging from 50 to 80 on the subscales of the HRQOL instrument, which indicates low to moderate function.

Yarbro and Ferrans (1998) used a mail survey to compare the QOL of 121 men receiving radiation (n = 53) and radical prostatectomy (n = 68) treatments for prostate cancer. The survey included the UCLA-PCI (Litwin et al., 1998) to assess physical function in terms of sexual, urinary and bowel symptoms. The Quality of Life Inventory (QLI) (Ferrans & Powers, 1985), based on Ferran's original work and the more recent Ferran's QOL conceptual model (1996) was used to measure well-being.

Subjects were identified through the cancer registries of a community cancer center and a teaching hospital. Of the total sample, 97% were Caucasian and 93% were married and living with a spouse or partner. Fifty-four percent of the sample had an annual household income of between $20,000 to $50,000, and 55% had a high school education. The mean age of the radical prostatectomy group was 68.6, and the mean age of the radiation group was 75.5. Approximately 75% of the total group was retired.

The results of the study showed no statistically significant differences in overall QOL between the two treatment groups. Furthermore, no differences were seen between treatment groups on well-being as measured by the QLI. Of a total of 30 possible points, men who received radical prostatectomy scored 23.85 on the QLI, and men who received radiation treatment scored 24.79.

Significant differences were seen between groups on the urinary and bowel function scales of the UCLA-PCI. The radiation group had better urinary function than the surgery group, whereas bowel function was better in the surgery group than in the radiation group. Sexual function was found to be poor in both groups.

Using a prospective, repeated measure, patient-report design, Talcott and associates (1998) studied 279 patients with newly diagnosed early stage prostate cancer that self-selected to radiation therapy ($N = 135$) or prostate surgery ($N = 125$) at one of several Harvard-affiliated medical centers. Patients that consented to participate in the study were sent a questionnaire prior to initiation of cancer therapy, at 3 months, and at 12 months after therapy initiation. Four instruments including a clinical abstraction form from the American College of Surgeon's Patterns of Care Study, patient questionnaires that addressed symptoms and quality of life, clinical data abstracted from a chart review, and a measure of comorbidity—the Index of Coexistent Disease (ICED)—were used.

Overall, radiation patients were slightly older (68 vs. 62 years) and had greater comorbidity, however, few patients were symptomatic from their comorbid disease. Pretreatment PSAs were nearly identical in both groups, as were clinical stage and tumor differentiation. Pretreatment symptoms of any kind were infrequent in both groups with the radiation group reporting slightly more symptoms of urinary frequency and impotence.

At three months after treatment, radiotherapy patients had symptoms of bowel urgency and diarrhea, which subsided by 12 months. Prostatectomy patients did not report bowel symptoms.

Daytime urinary frequency was more common at three months posttreatment than pretreatment in both treatment groups. However 58% of postprostatectomy patients reported urinary incontinence (UI) at 3 months and 35% had UI at 12 months (as measured by pad use) as compared to 5% at both 3 and 12 months in the radiotherapy group. While this study did demonstrate greater incidence of UI in men postprostatectomies than other previous series, the instrument used to measure incontinence may not have been sensitive to the extent of the problem as it currently exists. The authors reported that the number of absorbent pads used or use of penile clamp measured UI. In a recent study of UI in postprostatectomy men (Palmer et al., in press) of whom 70% leaked urine, results indicated that only half of the men studied ($N = 111$) used absorptive pads and 5% used penile clamps to manage their UI. This discrepancy in incidence raises the issue about the sensitivity of the instruments used to measure UI in this study.

Inadequate erections were present in one third of men pretreatment. Impotence was present in both treatment cohorts, however, postprostatectomy patients had a much higher incidence of incomplete erections. Both groups noted little improvement from 3 to 12 months. The small percentage of men who did note improvement was less than 65 years old.

Radiotherapy patients reported diarrhea, rectal urgency, and daytime urinary frequency in approximately one fourth of the patients, subsiding somewhat by 12 months. At 12 months 11% of postprostatectomy patients reported urinary incontinence and 35% used pads, while fewer radiotherapy patients reported incontinence or use of pads. In addition, those radiotherapy patients that reported incontinence and pad use were older than 65.

Strengths of this study were its prospective design, the inclusion of similar sample sizes in both groups, relatively little comorbidity in both groups, and the use of treatment facilities within the same health care system that provided the same state-of-the-art care. Data were collected at the key points as designated in the literature (i.e., symptoms are often most severe at 3 months postintervention and severely drop off by 1 year). Of note is that originally patients that received watchful waiting treatment were recruited, but numbers were so small that they were not included in the analysis. To assess whether nerve-sparing procedures were attempted or completed in the prostatectomy patients, a group of urologists, who were independent of the study and had not participated in the surgeries, reviewed the medical records of all patients in that cohort and made the determination whether nerve-sparing procedures had been completed. This provided triangulation of data collection that offered further strength to the design.

The use of the ICED strengthened the assessment of the impact of comorbid disease. The information that was provided suggested that the QOL instrument was used to ascertain information regarding symptoms and QOL. It did not discuss inclusion of global QOL or other aspects of the construct. Although QOL was identified as a variable to be included in the study, it was not reported as an outcome variable.

Overall, the article had much methodological strength and makes a contribution to the literature that is a significant improvement on previous work in this area. However, it provides continued evidence that symptoms of cancer therapy in general, and of prostate cancer treatment specifically, warrant further study to illuminate the nature of the symptoms that patients experience and the impact that they have on QOL. Specific attention to inclusion of instruments that are sensitive to measuring outcome variables should be a focus of future studies.

Fowler and colleagues (1993) predicted complications of 757 Medicare patients who underwent radical prostatectomy, and found some 47% of survey respondents noted daily leaking and some 31% required the use of pads, adult diapers, or penile clamps to manage wetness.

The prevalence of UI found in this study was further supported by a recent longitudinal study of 1291 community-based unselected men treated with radical prostatectomy (Stanford et al., 2000). At 6 months 20.5% had total urinary control, 45.6% had occasional leaking, 16.9% had frequent leakage, and 5.4% had no control. At 12 months, those with total control increased to 31%, while virtually the same number (43%) that noted occasional leaking at 6 months also leaked occasionally, and 10.9% and 2.8%, respectively, had frequent leakage and no control. Further, urodynamic studies of men with postprostactectomy UI correlated sphincter deficiency with subjective symptoms of stress incontinence, the type of incontinence most often seen postprostatectomy (Ficazzola & Nitti, 1998).

Summary and Conclusions

Researchers do not know the exact etiological mechanism of prostate cancer, though important progress in the treatment of prostate cancer in the past two decades has resulted in 5-year survival rates of 89% and 10-year survival rates of 63% (ACS, 2001). This dramatic progress in prostate cancer treatment is in sharp contrast to the understanding of the significant morbidity that regularly accompanies treatment. Although the impact that these effects of treatment may have on quality of life has been studied, study outcomes have been influenced by multiple design characteristics, including small sample sizes, use of cross-sectional designs which examine outcomes at one point in time, selecting patients treated at major tertiary referral centers or from a particular health plan, exclusion of certain age or ethnic groups, and so forth (Litwin et al., 1998).

Men treated for prostate cancer frequently feel ill-informed and unprepared to respond to the abrupt physical changes they face postprostatectomy (Moore & Estay, 1999). In a recent study examining the variation in men's long-term regret after treatment for metastatic prostate cancer, Clark, Wray, and Ashton (2001) found that regret was substantial and was associated with uncertainty about their disease, the quality of the treatment decisions in which they participated, and their QOL. These researchers found that regretful men had poorer scores on every measure of global and prostate-specific quality of life.

Although concern for the QOL has undoubtedly been pondered for some time, it is only over the last several decades that research has been engaged to attempt to define, measure, and capture the essence of this ambiguous concept. The attempts to define the concept are vast. However, due the personal nature of QOL, there continues to be a lack of consensus on its definition. A prevalent theme derived from the review of literature is that no one definition of QOL exists for all people. The QOL of individuals must be understood for nursing care to be effectively provided.

Studies aimed at determining common concerns of individuals by looking at various disease states have emerged as a way to guide clinicians toward evaluating and intervening to promote QOL. In addition, the multidimensional attribute of QOL has been the subject of several conceptual models. By evaluating individual domains, individual QOL values will become clearer.

Knowledge regarding the importance of QOL to individual patients facing monumental decisions regarding illness, treatment, and end of life is essential. Attempts toward understanding what constitutes quality of life have been made by researchers.

The measurement of QOL provides education to individual patients, informs and facilitates medical decision making, provides the defining issue if treatments are otherwise equivalent, and helps determine whether the goals of treatment have been met (Litwin, 1999; Wu & Cagney, 1996). These important clinical outcomes have elevated the construct of quality of life to an outcome measure of significant consequence in clinical research. Given the magnitude of prostate cancer in our society and the comparative lack of attention to the morbidity of prostate cancer treatment, the identification of factors influencing the QOL of patients with the disease is essential. This will lead to the development of nursing interventions aimed at helping individuals cope with the impact of disease on multiple dimensions of life and the ultimate goal—enhancing quality of life.

6

Nursing Care for Radical Prostatectomy

Penny Marschke

Radical prostatectomy plays a role in the treatment of those patients with cancer confined to the prostate. This chapter will focus on the nursing care associated with hospitalization, discharge planning, and possible long-term complications of patients undergoing radical prostatectomy.

The term radical prostatectomy can actually refer to three different surgical procedures designed to treat prostate cancer: the anatomic, radical retropubic prostatectomy; the perineal prostatectomy; and the laparoscopic prostatectomy. A brief description of these surgeries will aid in the appreciation and understanding of patient's postoperative needs. Each of these approaches, to some degree, carries the side effects of urinary incontinence and erectile dysfunction. The goals of prostatectomy, regardless of surgical approach, are: (1) cancer control by removing all the visible tumor, (2) the preservation of urinary continence, and (3) the preservation of erectile function.

RADICAL PROSTATECTOMY TREATMENT OPTIONS

The anatomic, radical retropubic prostatectomy involves removing the prostate with controlled hemostasis and clear visualization of the neurovascular bundles that innervate the corpora cavernosa of the penis (Catalona, Ramos, & Carvahal, 1999). Using either spinal or epidural anesthesia, the surgery begins with an incision that extends from the umbilicus to the pubis (Walsh, 1998). Initially, a staging lymphadenectomy is performed to determine if the lymph nodes are cancer free. If so, the surgery continues (Walsh, 1998). This surgery involves maintaining a bloodless field while removing the prostate gland and all visible cancer cells without damaging the urethral sphincter responsible for urinary continence or the neurovascular bundles located on both sides of the prostate responsible for erections (Walsh, 1998). To ensure cancer control, occasionally, it may be necessary to remove one or both neurovascular bundles. Once the prostate gland, seminal vesicles and vas deferens are removed, the bladder neck is reconstructed and anastomosed to the urethra (Walsh, 1998). Two pelvic drains are placed for approximately three days to evacuate any urine leaking from the anastomosis (Walsh, 1998). An indwelling catheter is inserted during surgery and remains in place for 10 to 21 days to allow the reconstructed urinary tract to heal (DeMarco, Bihrle, & Foster, 2000; Santis, Hoffman, & Wolf, 2000; Walsh, 1998). Generally, the patient can be discharged from the hospital on the third postoperative day (Gardner et al., 2000).

The perineal prostatectomy is performed under epidural or spinal anesthesia by making an incision from one ischial tuberosity to the other with the apex of the incision approximately 1.5 cm above the anus (Gibbons, 1998). The prostate is teased away from the rectum, bladder, urethra, and vas deferens (Gibbons, 1998). The seminal vesicles are removed with the prostate and then the urethra is anastomosed to the anterior bladder neck. A penrose drain is placed on each side of the anastomosis and an indwelling catheter is placed and taped to the midline of the abdomen (Gibbons, 1998). The patient can be discharged on the second postoperative day (Weldon, Tavel, & Newirth, 1997). In patients, identified as high risk prior to the perineal prostatectomy, an open or laparoscopic lymph node dissection is performed to identify positive nodes that would indicate that cancer has spread outside of the prostatic capsule (Gibbons, 1998).

The newest approach being explored is the laparoscopic prostatectomy which is performed under general anesthesia. First a 12 mm trocar is placed through a minilaporotomy just below the umbilicus (Abbou et al., 2000). As insufflation, the process of injecting carbon dioxide into the peritoneum to achieve exposure during laparoscopic surgery, is begun, the secondary trocars are placed under visual control. Through the trocars, visualization of the field (including the neurovascular bundles) is maintained. The prostate gland is dissected out and removed in an endobag® through the umbilical port site (Abbou et al., 2000). The bladder neck is anastomosed to the urethra and an indwelling catheter is inserted into the bladder. A small suction-drain is inserted and left in place for 48 hours (Abbou et al., 2000). Depending on the experience level of the surgeon, this surgery can take from 7 hours without lymphadenectomy to 8.6 hours with lymphadenectomy (Abbou et al., 2000; Guilloneau & Vallancien, 2000; Jacob et al., 2000).

Each of these surgical approaches to treating organ-confined prostate cancer has its advantages and disadvantages which must be weighed by the patient, his family, and the urologist. The major advantage of the anatomic, radical retropubic prostatectomy is that the surgeon can visualize the entire surgical field, therefore allowing for more precise dissection of tissue.

The major advantage of the perineal prostatectomy is less blood loss because the dorsal vein complex is not removed with the prostate. However, this also means surgeons are not able to remove as much tissue therefore, positive surgical margins are more likely in men who have capsular penetration (Walsh & Worthington, 1995). Compared to the anatomic, retropubic radical prostatectomy, the incidence for postoperative complications of erectile dysfunction and rectal injury are also greater in patients who undergo a perineal prostatectomy (Klimaszewski & Karlowicz, 1995; Lassen & Kearse, 1995). Despite the limitations, the perineal approach has seen a recent resurgence in its popularity because of the trend toward minimally invasive surgery and a focus on reducing the morbidity and hospital stay of patients (Hewitt, 2001).

The major advantage of the laparoscopic approach is that it is minimally invasive. Therefore, in theory, patients should be able to return to activities of daily living earlier than those who undergo an open approach. However, because this approach is rarely used in the United States, the data are too preliminary to make any meaningful comparisons in terms of urinary incontinence, erectile dysfunction, or cancer control.

Knowledge of how each of the surgeries is performed and the advantages and disadvantages of each also helps nurses to identify the patient's postoperative needs. For example, in each of the approaches, discernibly, the anastomosis of the urethra to the bladder neck must be protected. Therefore, catheter care is of upmost importance. Likewise, for all of the surgical approaches the proximity of the rectal wall to the surgical site renders that area in need of special attention. That is, no rectal procedures should be performed postoperatively. Additional nursing interventions to promote comfort, facilitate urinary elimination, support wound healing, maintain fluid and electrolyte balance, and prevent possible complications such as thrombophlebitis and pulmonary embolism also need to be addressed (Klimaszewski & Karlowicz, 1995).

NURSING CARE DURING HOSPITALIZATION

Since the radical retropubic prostatectomy is the most widely performed procedure, general wound and catheter care, fluid and electrolyte management, pain management, and the prevention of complications will be addressed. Each and every physician, as well as institution has their specific postoperative orders that are to be followed for their radical retropubic prostatectomy patients. The approach to nursing care that will be discussed is that which is followed at The Johns Hopkins Hospital regarded as one the Centers of Excellence for Prostate Cancer by the National Cancer Institute.

Wound Care

Wound care consists mainly of assessing and observing the surgical incision for signs of healing as well as signs of infection. The closed suction drains which usually ooze a serous, blood-tinged fluid are left in place until they cease to function (Walsh, 1998). Usually, the drains and staples are removed on the day of discharge. The surgical site is covered with steri-strips which eventually peel off as they loosen in approximately one to two weeks.

Catheter Care

Urinary elimination consists mainly of maintaining a closed urethral catheter drainage system (Klimaszewski & Karlowicz, 1995). Since the indwelling catheter acts as a splint for the urethral anastomosis at the bladder neck, the focus of all precautions is to protect the catheter from becoming dislodged or removed. Also, the entire urinary drainage system must be cared for in such a manner as to protect it from the possibility of infection; that is, the drainage bag cannot drag on the floor, and each port of the system should be wiped with alcohol before and after opening it. To promote adequate drainage and avoid excessive manipulation, the catheter should be secured to the patient's thigh with excess tubing coiled on the bed. The drainage bag should be affixed below bladder level (Klimaszewski & Karlowicz, 1995). Assessing and observing the urinary drainage for amount, color, and consistency is important. Bleeding is common for the first 24 hours following surgery; however, excessive or continued bleeding or the presence of clots should be reported to the urologist (Klimaszewski & Karlowicz, 1995). Gentle, manual irrigation of the catheter may be ordered by the urologist to restore a patent catheter system. Patients are discharged with the indwelling catheter in place. The catheter will remain in place for 10 to 21 days to allow the reconstructed urinary tract to heal (DeMarco, Bihrle, & Foster, 2000; DeWolf, 2000; Walsh, 1998).

Fluids and Electrolyte Management

Due the possibility of excessive blood loss intraoperatively, many patients donate two to three autologous units of blood prior to the surgery. Intravenous fluids are administered for the first 48 hours postoperatively or until the patient is tolerating a liquid diet. Unless it is medically contraindicated, a fluid intake of 2,500 to 3,000 cc/day is desired (Klimaszewski & Karlowicz, 1995). Because of possible fluid shifts, patients must be monitored carefully prior to ambulation. The patient should be allowed and encouraged to dangle his lower extremities prior to standing and walking.

Pain Management

Pain associated with the incision is managed with intravenous patient-controlled analgesia (PCA) using morphine. Walsh (1998) reported that if pain control is not adequate, intravenous ketorolac tromethamine can also be used; this combination of analgesic agents reduces the risk of postoperative ileus. The goal of pain management is to keep the patient's perception of pain at or below three on a scale of one to ten (with one being minimal/no discomfort). Klimaszewski and Karlowicz (1995) note that antispasmodics such as oxybutynin chloride (Ditropan®) and propantheline bromide (Pro-Banthine®) may be administered to relieve painful bladder spasms that result when receptors in the bladder wall are stimulated to cause involuntary bladder contractions. For a further discussion of pain assessment and management, see chapter 11.

Prevention of Complications

The most worrisome postoperative complications in this population are the possibility of thrombophlebitis and pulmonary embolism. To prevent the occurrence of these complications the patient must ambulate with assistance the first day after surgery a minimum of four times; complete dorsiflexion exercises 100 times every hour while awake; use the incentive spirometer 10 times every hour while awake; turn, cough, and deep breathe every hour while awake; and wear TED® stockings in addition to sequential compression devices. Patients are not permitted to sit. Patients may recline in a chair with their feet and legs above their heart level (Walsh & Worthington, 1995).

The general concerns that nurses must be aware of while caring for the radical retropubic prostatectomy patient were reviewed. The specific interventions necessary to care for patients with a history of heart disease, deep vein thrombosis, and/or diabetes should be tailored on an individual basis.

DISCHARGE PLANNING
(FIRST 6 WEEKS AFTER SURGERY)

This section will cover discharge planning that is pertinent to the radical retropubic prostatectomy patient. Even though the standard discharge instructions for a surgical patient apply, for example, call your physician for a temperature greater than 101°F; no lifting greater than 10 pounds, these will not be reviewed in the chapter.

A study by Moore and Estey (1999) revealed that at discharge, the radical prostatectomy patients felt there were many knowledge gaps regarding catheter care, postoperative pain, incontinence, and erectile dysfunction. These identified areas of patient concern, plus other serious postoperative complications, will be discussed.

Postoperative Complications

Even after discharge from the hospital, the greatest worry and concern to the medical community for this group of surgical patients remains the possible development of a deep venous thrombosis or a pulmonary embolism. Therefore, before leaving the hospital, the patients must know and be able to recognize the signs and symptoms of a deep vein thrombosis and a pulmonary embolism. Walsh and Worthington (1995) have noted that blood clots in the legs can occur in as many as 12% and pulmonary embolism can occur in an estimated 2% to 5% of men after radical prostatectomy. Patients should be aware and call their urologist if they experience any pain in the calf of their legs or swelling in their ankles or legs. Patients should be aware that these clots may break loose and travel to the lung producing a life-threatening condition known as a pulmonary embolus. However, a pulmonary embolus can occur even in the absence of pain or swelling in their leg. The signs and symptoms of a pulmonary embolus can include chest pain (especially when taking a deep breath), shortness of breath, syncope, and/or hemoptosis (Smith, Britt, & Terry, 1995). If patients develop any of these signs or symptoms they should be instructed to go to their closest emergency room and state that they need to be evaluated for deep venous thrombosis or pulmonary embolus. Doppler ultrasound can be used to evaluate the leg veins for clots and a spiral CT of the lungs can diagnose a pulmonary embolus. If the diagnosis is made early, treatment with anticoagulation is effective (Smith, Britt, & Terry, 1995).

Patients should be instructed to observe and assess their surgical incisions on a daily basis. The best time is before a shower. For the first week at home, the patient should be instructed to cover his surgical incision with a protective plastic wrap (e.g., Saran Wrap) so as to ensure that the steri-strips® will remain in place for at least one week before naturally loosening. Patients should be taught to look for drainage from the wound. This can be manifested as a clear, serous fluid or blood and pus. In either case, the patient should know to call his urologist.

Patients should also be aware of the fact that urinary tract infections are not uncommon following prolonged use of a catheter. Signs and symptoms are cloudy or foul smelling urine or purulent drainage from around the catheter. In either case, the patient should know which symptoms warrant a call to his urologist and an antibiotic will be prescribed.

Catheter Care and Urinary Continence

Before leaving the hospital, the patient must be instructed on how to care for his indwelling catheter including meatal care, leg bag care, and night bag care. In addition, the patient needs to understand what to expect when the catheter is removed, and how he will progress toward regaining his urinary continence. Initially, when the catheter is removed, the patient can expect to experience such irritative voiding symptoms as urgency and stress incontinence. Walsh and Worthington (1995) described how urinary control generally returns in three phases. Phase One—the patient is dry when lying down at night. Phase Two—he will be dry when walking around and Phase Three—the patient is dry when he stands up after sitting.

In 2000, Marschke noted in a study of 51 radical prostatectomy patients that by 6 months post-op, 67% reported that they were completely dry and requiring no pads; 27% experienced mild incontinence requiring 1 or fewer pads/24 hours and only 6% were experiencing moderate incontinence requiring >1 pad/24 hours. Many varieties of pads/diapers and padded underwear are available for use until the urinary control returns. Walsh and Worthington (1995) express the need to tell the patient never to wear an incontinence device with an attached bag, a condom catheter or clamp because they will never develop the muscle control needed to be continent.

Wei, Dunn, Marcovich, Montie, and Sanda (2000) reported that the significant predictors of continence outcome in the radical retropubic prostatectomy were preoperative continence, patient age, and nerve-sparing approach. Joseph (2001) states that one of the most common postprostatectomy continence problems is stress urinary incontinence caused by an incompetent external sphincter due to nerve injury during surgery or inadequate healing. Pelvic muscle exercises, for example, Kegel exercises, can be done by the patient to help strengthen the external sphincter (Walsh & Worthington, 1995). Walsh and Worthington (1995) recommend that once, during each void, the patient should completely stop his urinary stream by contracting the muscles in his buttocks. They also advise that the patient should be informed not to do Kegel exercises at other times because that will tire the sphincter muscle.

Postoperative Pain Management

The majority of postoperative pain is associated with bladder spasms. They are painful, uncontrollable contractions of the bladder. Usually they are strong enough to force urine out of the bladder and around the catheter. Bladder spasms are caused by the presence of the catheter and should subside once the catheter is removed. Just as when there is a piece of dirt in your eye, it is only natural for the eye to blink; likewise the bladder will occasionally "blink" or spasm until the catheter is removed.

Erectile Function

For erectile function, patients need to know that erections will return gradually. Determinants of erectile function after surgery include: preoperative erectile function, age of the patient, clinical and pathological stage of the disease, and surgical technique (Quinlan, Epstein, & Carter, 1991; Rabbani, Stapleton, & Kattan, 2000). Walsh and Worthington (1995) note that the major stimulus for erections during the first year postoperatively is tactile sensation. For this reason they suggest that patients experiment with sexual activity but not until six weeks after surgery to be sure that everything is well healed. Three months postoperatively, some urologists will give those patients who are candidates for taking sildenafil citrate the option of trying the drug. However, Zippe and colleagues (2000) stress that successful treatment of erectile dysfunction with sildenafil citrate after radical prostatectomy depends on the presence of the neurovascular bundles. Their data also suggests that the response to sildenafil citrate is not related to the time interval between the surgery and initiation of the drug therapy but is related to the dose of the sildenafil citrate.

LONG-TERM COMPLICATIONS

Some of the long-term complications that can occur after radical prostatectomy include bladder neck contracture, total incontinence, erectile dysfunction, or a rising PSA. Between 3% and 12% of men after radical prostatectomy will develop a constriction of the bladder neck, usually a result of scar tissue around the bladder neck (Walsh & Worthington, 1995). The symptom is a dribbling urinary stream, which is sometimes difficult to differentiate from the moderate incontinence that often occurs after a radical prostatectomy. Borboroglu, Sands, Roberts, and Amling (2000) found that several comorbidities associated with microvascular disease are significant risk factors for the development of bladder neck contracture after radical prostatectomy. These comorbidities included coronary artery disease, diabetes mellitus, hypertension, cerebral vascular accident and chronic obstructive pulmonary disease. A strong predictor is current cigarette smoking. The authors also noted that transurethral dilation and transurethral incision are equally effective as initial treatment of bladder neck contracture.

Urinary Incontinence

In the majority of cases, urinary continence improves over time for the radical prostatectomy patient. In the extremely rare case when this does not occur, a cystometrogram (CMG) is completed to determine the urinary bladder pressure at various volumes of fluid. If incontinence persists for more than a year, or is severe, one option for treatment is an artificial urinary sphincter prosthesis. Barrett and Licht (1998) suggest that unless contraindicated, patients should have had a trial of anticholinergic and/or alpha-sympathomimetic medication along with pelvic floor exercises before considering the surgical placement of an artificial sphincter. The artificial sphincter is a small implanted device which works by shifting sterile fluid in and out of three main components of this closed system. Under general anesthesia, the cuff is placed around the bladder neck or bulbar urethra, the control pump mechanism is implanted in the scrotum and the reservoir is placed in the lower abdomen. Within six to eight weeks after surgery, the patients are usually ready to learn how to activate the sphincter device. The patient will learn that when the cuff is filled with fluid, it gently holds the urethra closed to keep urine in the bladder. When the pump (located in the scrotum) is squeezed and released, this opens the cuff. As the fluid flows out of the cuff and into the reservoir (located in the abdomen), the empty cuff allows urine to flow out of the bladder. Several minutes after the bladder has emptied, the fluid will automatically flow from the reservoir back into the cuff, causing the urethra to be held closed again. Patients will also learn when to deactivate their artificial sphincter—for example, those needing to intermittently self-catheterize or those patients who are dry at night can deactivate the device during sleep.

Permanent restrictions for artificial sphincter patients include riding a bicycle or exercise bike with a standard saddle seat, and horseback riding (Barrett & Licht, 1998). Also, the patient should be aware that he will continue to be incontinent during his surgical recovery until the sphincter is activated. During that time period, the use of penile clamps should be discouraged. Postoperative complications can include infection, mechanical malfunction, cuff erosion, hematoma, and retention.

Erectile Dysfunction

One of the first pieces of information needed to help in discerning erectile dysfunction after radical prostatectomy is how many cavernosal nerves were spared during the procedure. Patients who have undergone a nonnerve-sparing procedure (the nerves were removed during surgery) will not respond to sildenafil citrate postoperatively. Feng, Huang, Kaptein, Kaswick, and Aboseif (2000) have found that sildenafil citrate® is an equally effective treatment for erectile dysfunction after bilateral and unilateral nerve-sparing procedures. All of the patients in this study received 25 to 100 mg of sildenafil citrate in a flexible dose escalation schedule.

One of the simplest approaches to assisting with erectile dysfunction can involve placing a band (e.g., Actis ring, ponytail holder, Coban®) around the base of the penis prior to foreplay. This will assist those men who experience venous leak. Venous leak results from lack of venous compression. Meredith (1995) explains that the blood flowing into the arteries may be sufficient to achieve an erection, but there is not enough pressure exerted on the veins to compress them and prevent the blood from leaving the area.

Other options available for treatment include intracorporeal injection therapy, vacuum erection devices, and penile prostheses. The penile prosthesis is usually considered as the last form of treatment since it does involve surgery.

Intracorporeal injection therapy involves having the patient inject the smallest amount of drug needed to produce an erection strong enough for vaginal penetration, yet subsiding prior to the development of priapism. Medications that can be used include papaverine, phentolamine, and Prostaglandin®. An erection lasting less than 30 minutes is considered inadequate, whereas an erection lasting longer than two and a half hours, known as priapism, is approaching the uncomfortable stage (Meredith, 1995, p. 353). An additional caveat is limiting the number of injections per week to reduce the possibility of developing fibrosis.

The vacuum erection device (VED) is designed to create an erection through the use of suction. Meredith (1995) describes the use of the VED as follows: A well-lubricated cylinder with a penile ring at the base is placed over the penis. Suction is applied to create a vacuum in the cylinder. Once an erection is achieved, the penile ring is slipped down onto the base of the penis, trapping blood in the corporeal bodies. The cylinder is removed and the man is ready to engage in sexual activity. Caution should be exercised to remove the ring within 30 to 40 minutes after engaging it to avoid tissue damage. Ganem, Lucey, Janosko, and Carson (1998) reported that, when used correctly, VEDs carry low morbidity and few recognized complications.

Penile prostheses are available in two varieties: (1) the rigid or semirigid; and (2) the inflatable. Each type carries its own advantages and disadvantages. All of the risks and benefits need to be discussed in thorough detail with the patient before he and his partner decide which variety will best fit their life style and needs. Meredith (1995) describes the surgical procedure: all of the penile implants are inserted into the spongy tissue of the penis (corpora cavernosa) that fills with blood, the space normally occupied with blood can be used for the implant instead.

Regarding the actual devices the semirigid rods are made of silicone and may have a flexible metal core that allows the patient to bend his penis down and fit it comfortably and inconspicuously into his underwear (Meredith, 1995). The inflatable prosthesis which most closely resembles a natural erection consists of two hollow cylinders that are positioned in the penis; a pump and valve system that is placed into the scrotum, and a reservoir of sterile liquid that is stationed in the lower abdomen (Meredith, 1995, p. 349). Squeezing the pump will activate the cylinders to fill, thus creating an erection. Carson, Mulcahy, and Govier (2000) performed a long-term study of the American Medical Systems 700CX three-piece inflatable penile prostheses, focusing on longevity, morbidity, and patient satisfaction. The median follow-up for this group of patients was 47.7 months. The researchers found that in the majority of men, the penile prosthesis produced suitable erections and excellent patient satisfaction. They also commented that the implant reliability was excellent and that the postoperative morbidity was low.

Rising PSA

The PSA should be undectable (< 0.1) after a radical prostatectomy. A DRE is not needed as long as the PSA remains undectable. A rise in the PSA postoperatively can be very distressing for the patient since this evidence of a biochemical recurrence usually signifies that the cancer was not completely eliminated. Pound and associates (1999) note that while removing the prostate gland successfully eradicates the disease in about 60% to 70% of men, in about one-third of the patients, the cancer is not completely eliminated and the PSA levels begin to rise within 10 years following surgery. By studying the natural history of progression for PSA elevation following radical prostatectomy in nearly 2000 men; Pound and colleagues (1999) found that these men remained disease free an average of eight years and lived an average of five years after metastatic disease was confirmed by radionuclide bone scan, chest radiograph, or other body imaging.

This chapter has reviewed the surgical approaches to radical prostatectomy as well as the necessary nursing care during hospitalization and for discharge planning. Likewise some of the long-term outcomes of the surgery such as bladder neck contracture, urinary incontinence and erectile dysfunction were discussed. The lack of nursing research is very evident within this area of prostate cancer literature. Most of the articles and research to date have been concentrated within the areas of screening and advanced prostate cancer. A dire need exists for research within the area of nursing care for this group of patients.

7
Nursing Care for Radiation Treatment

Vanna M. Dest

The role of radiation therapy (RT) in the treatment of prostate cancer has come to the forefront over the past 15 years with various advances in the field of radiation oncology. As a result, the assessment and management of acute and chronic side effects of treatment, patient and family education, and addressing psychosocial issues such as sexuality and body image have become major aspects of care that nurses provide. This chapter will address and review the nursing care of the patient receiving RT for prostate cancer.

RADIATION THERAPY TREATMENT OPTIONS FOR PROSTATE CANCER

Treatment options in RT include external beam therapy, brachytherapy, or a combination of both. Treatment decisions are based upon various prognostic factors. These factors include extent of tumor, prostate specific antigen (PSA) level, and histologic grade of tumor or Gleason score. Other factors that must be considered include age of patient, existing medical problems, clinical morbidity, and patient preference. It has been postulated that the pretreatment PSA is the strongest independent predictor of treatment outcome after radiation therapy (Hanks & Horowitz, 2000).

Various approaches are used to select the most appropriate treatment plan for patients with prostate cancer. Partin and colleagues (1997) looked at data from three academic institutions and developed a nonogram analyzing pretreatment factors predictive of extraprostatic disease.

These factors included serum PSA level, clinical stage, and Gleason score, which can be used to determine the risk of lymph node involvement, seminal vesicle involvement, and extracapsular disease in men with carcinoma of the prostate gland.

The American Brachytherapy Society (ABS) recommends that men with T1 to T2a disease, PSA level < 10 ng/ml, and Gleason score less than or equal to 6 are good candidates for brachytherapy alone. However, men may choose to solely opt for external beam RT. Patients with stage T2c or higher disease, PSA levels > 20 ng/ml, or Gleason scores of 8 to 10 should receive combined modality of external beam RT, brachytherapy, and hormonal therapy. Patients falling between these parameters must be evaluated for perineural invasion, multiple positive biopsies, and tumor location. The treatment plan for those patients may require combined external beam RT with or without the administration of hormonal therapy (Nag, Beyer, Friedland, Grimm, & Nath, 1999). The use of hormonal therapy is also indicated in men with advanced prostate carcinoma. (See chapter 1 for Staging Classification.)

Ragde, Grado, Nadir, and Elgamal (2000) have developed another approach. They recommend the utilization of brachytherapy alone for patients with Gleason scores < 7, PSA levels less than or equal to 10 ng/ml, and nonpalpable or small solitary lesions < 2.0 centimeters in diameter. For patients with Gleason scores of 7 or greater, PSA levels greater than 10 ng/ml, or nodules greater than 2.0 centimeters in size, the risk of extraprostatic disease increases. Therefore, the combined modality of external beam RT and brachytherapy are utilized. For patients with high-risk disease, neoadjuvant or adjuvant hormonal therapy may be added.

EXTERNAL BEAM RADIATION

External beam RT is delivered by a linear accelerator, which emits radiation in the form of x-rays. It is typically delivered five days a week (i.e., Monday through Friday). The treatment is painless and generally takes less than two minutes to deliver. It commonly takes longer to set up the treatment than it takes for the patients to receive it. Patients are not radioactive when receiving external beam RT because the source of radiation is outside their body.

The planning of radiation to the pelvic area differs in terms of technique used, also called the simulation. The conventional setup is called the four-field or box technique, which directs the radiation at anterior/posterior and posterior/anterior (AP/PA) fields and two lateral fields. The simulation consists of mapping out the area that needs to be treated and takes up to 60 minutes to complete. Patients are in the supine position and usually require rectal and bladder contrast to aid in localization of the prostate. computed tomography (CT)-based treatment planning is not used and treatment field size is determined by bony landmarks and not target volumes. The total dose of radiation using conventional setup ranges from 64 to 70 Gray (Gy) over a period of 6 to 8 weeks (Chao, Perez, & Brady, 1999). This conventional setup is not routinely utilized since the advent of three-dimensional conformal radiation therapy.

The three-dimensional conformal radiation therapy (3DCRT) is the process by which a radiation dose is planned and delivered to a target volume and less radiation to adjacent normal structures, such as the bladder and rectum. The setup for 3DCRT involves immobilization of the patient with the utilization of posterior body cast and obtaining a CAT scan of the pelvis so that the prostate gland is reconstructed in three dimensions by the treatment-planning computer. As a result, multiple beams are directed at the prostate gland, which is the target volume and minimal radiation to the adjacent structures. This allows for dose escalation and decreased morbidity due to side effects (Epstein & Hanks, 1992; Hanks & Horowitz, 2000). A recent study by Perez and associates (2000) found that 3DCRT spares normal tissue, delivers higher doses for longer disease-free survival and less morbidity. The total dose of radiation therapy delivered with 3DCRT ranges from 68 to 82 Gy (Hanks & Horowitz, 2000). This type of planning cures more prostate cancers causing fewer complications (Hanks, 2000). Institutions, such as Fox Chase Cancer Center and University of Michigan, have examined overall survival with the use of conventional versus 3DCRT for men with pretreatment PSA levels less than 10 ng/ml and those with pretreatment PSA between 10 to 20 ng/ml. They found that the use of 3DCRT improved 5-year survival by almost 30%, compared to conventional methods. Hanks (2000) feels strongly that this technique should be utilized universally amongst all radiation oncologists in the treatment-planning phase for men with prostate cancer.

The course of external beam RT ranges from five to eight weeks. Eight weeks of external beam radiation is given when utilized alone or five weeks of external beam irradiation when preceded or followed by brachytherapy boost. With combined modality, the total dose of external RT ranges from 40 to 50 Gy over a period of five weeks (Nag et al., 1999).

SEED IMPLANTATION/BRACHYTHERAPY

Seed implantation, also called brachytherapy, can be used alone or in conjunction with external beam irradiation. This technique of seed implantation allows for the delivery of a high dose of radiation to the prostate while sparing most of the adjacent structures, the bladder and rectum. Although seed implantation has been used for many years, the past 15 years have seen this technique perfected. The ultrasound-guided transperineal technique was developed by Holm and colleagues (1983) and was further tested by Blasko, Ragde, and Grimm (1991), who performed the first procedure at Northwest Hospital in Seattle, Washington. The purpose of this technique is to assure proper placement of the needles, which house the radioactive seeds. The size and shape of the prostate gland determines the number of radioactive seeds implanted. The prostate volume size is an important factor in treatment planing and implant success. It is felt that the prostate volume should be less than 60 cm^3 for a successful implant to be done (Blasko, Grimm, Ragde, & Schumacher, 1997). The prostate volume is determined by a procedure called the volume study, which is accomplished by the use of transrectal ultrasonography. Images in 5-millimeter intervals are obtained of the prostate gland, extending from the base of the gland to the apex. It is important that patients undergo a bowel preparation the day before the procedure. For clarity of the ultrasound images, the rectum must be free of intestinal gas and feces. The bowel preparation may consist of clear liquid diet for 24 hours and the administration of an oral laxative such as Milk of Magnesia® the night before the study, Fleets® enemas the morning of the procedure, and antiflatulents containing simethicone such as Mylicon® or Gas-X®.

Another important factor with brachytherapy is evaluation of pubic arch interference. If a patient has a narrow pubic arch, it maybe infeasible to implant the entire gland due to interference from the symphysis pubis. Often times, patients may require the use of hormonal therapy to decrease the size of the prostate gland, counteract the pubic arch interference, or in the presence of high-risk disease. The medications used include Lupron depot® (leuprolide acetate) or Zoladex® (zoserlin acetate) in conjunction with Casodex® (bicalutamide) or Eulexin® (flutamide), to accomplish total androgen blockade. The course of therapy is approximately 3 to 6 months. Side effects commonly experienced with hormonal therapy include hot flashes, decreased libido, impotence, nausea, and diarrhea.

There are primarily two types of radioactive isotopes used for seed implantation in prostate cancer, Iodine 125 (I-125) and Palladium 103 (Pd-103). The difference between the two isotopes is their half-life. Half-life is defined as the period of time required for a radioactive isotope to lose half of its radioactivity. Iodine 125 has a half-life of 60 days, whereas Palladium 103 has a half-life of 17 days. Iodine seeds are most widely utilized in less aggressive cancers as they deliver a relatively low dose rate over a longer period of time. Palladium seeds are generally utilized for patients with more aggressive disease and associated with more intense urinary and rectal symptoms but for a lesser period of time than Iodine 125 (Merrick, Butler, Farthing, Dorsey, & Adamovich, 1998; Nath, Meigooni, & Melillo, 1992). Cha and colleagues (1999) investigated the utilization of Pd-103 and I-125 in a matched control group. They found no significant difference in survival rates in the patients receiving Pd-103 or I-125 seeds. In addition, they found that one isotope was not superior to the other.

Because the half-life of the two radioisotopes is so diverse, the duration and intensity of side effects varies. With Iodine 125, the seeds continue to emit radiation for a period of 20 months and then are considered to be inert. In contrast, Palladium 103 seeds emit radiation for a period of six months before they are considered inactive. Side effects with Pd-103 are more intense with a shorter duration in comparison to I-125. The American Brachytherapy Society (ABS) recommends that for patients being treated with brachytherapy alone, the prescription dose is 115-120 Gy for Pd-103 and 144 Gy for I-125. Patients with high risk disease are treated with combined external beam RT and brachytherapy. The ABS recommends the prescription dose for brachytherapy boost with Pd-103 range between 80 to 90 Gy and 100 to 110 Gy for I-125 (Nag et al., 1999).

Seed implantation is primarily done as an outpatient surgical procedure. Men are placed in dorsal lithotomy position during the 1- to 2-hour procedure, for which general, spinal, or local anesthesia is administered. An average of 25 to 40 temporary needles are inserted via ultrasound positioned template into the perineum of the patient (Abel et al., 1999; Cash & Dattoli, 1997). Each needle can house from one to six radioactive seeds, which is dependent upon pre-planning dosimetry. The average number of seeds implanted ranges from 100 to 150, each measuring 4.5 millimeters by 0.8 millimeters (Abel et al., 1999).

After implantation of radioactive seeds into the prostate gland, a cystourethroscopy is performed. This is done to evaluate for bleeding and to retrieve any seeds which may have been placed in or migrated to the bladder or urethra.

Postoperative Care of the Prostate Brachytherapy Patient

The focus of postoperative implant care is to establish stability of cardiovascular status, genitourinary status, skin integrity, and control of pain. The patient should be assessed for bleeding, drainage, edema and ecchymosis of perineal area. The ecchymosis and edema can extend up to the scrotum. Application of ice packs for the first 24 hours can minimize the degree of scrotal and perineal swelling, ecchymosis, and incidence of hematoma formation, which is caused by needle trauma. The occurrence of postoperative infection is rare, but patients are given prophylactic antibiotics (Abel et al., 1999).

If an indwelling urinary catheter is inserted during the perioperative phase, men may experience symptoms of urethritis. Therefore it is imperative for patients to urinate after the catheter is removed. Patients may also experience hematuria after seed implantation. This is caused by needle trauma to the bladder, urethra, and prostate gland. The hematuria generally subsides within 12 to 24 hours after implant, but may persist for up to two to three days. It is rare to see persistent hematuria or clots that require continuous bladder irrigation. However, as a precaution, patients are required to stop taking aspirin, aspirin-containing products, nonsteroidal anti-inflammatory drugs (NSAIDs), and anticoagulants prior to surgery. For patients on anticoagulation therapy, either Coumadin® is discontinued prior to surgery, if risk factors are minimal, or the use of Heparin IV or Lovenox® SC is indicated.

Patients are instructed not to perform any heavy lifting or strenuous activity for at least three days following surgery. Upon discharge, patients are generally prescribed a narcotic analgesic such as Vicodin® (hydrocodone & acetaminophen) or Percocet® (oxycodone & acetaminophen) to relieve discomfort associated with insertion of needles and the trauma it causes. Patients are also prescribed a broad spectrum antibiotic, such as Cipro® (ciprofloxacin) 500 mg BID for five to seven days, as a prophylaxis against infection. To decrease signs and symptoms of inflammation and edema, a steroid such as Medrol dosepak® is prescribed for 7 days. And lastly, patients are prescribed one of the alpha-adrenergic blockers, which include Cardura® (doxazosin), Hytrin® (terazosin), or Flomax® (tamsulosin). These drugs act by relaxing smooth muscle of the urinary sphincter, thereby decreasing obstructive and irritative symptoms related to implantation.

Even though a cystourethroscopy was performed during surgery, patients are instructed to strain their urine for seven days after implantation, for the passage of any radioactive seeds. If a seed is found, it is recommended that patients retrieve the seed with tweezers, put into a glass container, and return it to the Radiation Oncology department.

Radiation Safety Precautions with the Prostate Brachytherapy Patient

Safety is always a tremendous concern for patients and family members of those receiving brachytherapy. Patients that choose implant therapy have permanent seeds, which lose their radioactivity over a specific period of time. The radiation emitted by the radioactive seeds has weak penetration and the exposure to others and the general public is minimal (Smathers et al., 1999). Regardless, certain radiation precautions must be followed. Patients are advised not to have close physical contact with pregnant women and children under the age of six (i.e., having them sit on lap) for one half-life of the radioisotope. Therefore, patients receiving I-125 seeds should follow the above precautions for two months and for those receiving Pd-103, precautions should be exercised for 17 days or three weeks for simplicity (Nag et al., 1999). In addition, they should abstain from sexual intercourse for two weeks after implant and wear a condom during intercourse for at least one month or the first six times. Radioactive seeds are implanted in the seminal vesicles, which are the reservoir for semen and seminal fluid. Wearing a condom prevents the low probability of a seed being discharged into the vagina (Blasko, Grimm, Ragde, & Schumacher, 1997). Patient may also experience hematospermia, in which semen may be dark brown or bloody in color.

Assessment and Identification of Side Effects of Radiation Therapy

The role of the nurse in radiation oncology requires an understanding of the principles of radiotherapy and radiobiology with regard to its effect on cancer cells and normal cells, treatment side effects, and psychosocial issues related to treatment and the disease process. Patients need to be assessed and managed throughout the entire treatment process with close follow-up thereafter. Side effects of RT can be divided into acute and chronic or early and late side effects. Acute or early side effects of RT occur in rapidly dividing cells or those in cell division. These side effects occur during RT and can last from 1 to 6 months after therapy is completed. The presence of acute side effects does not predict the occurrence of late or chronic side effects. Late or chronic effects of radiation therapy occur in slowly proliferating cells, such as fibroblasts, endothelial, or parenchymal stem cells. Often times the full effect of radiation may not be apparent for months to years after therapy is completed. Chronic effects are usually a result of damage to microcirculation or vasculature. Chronic side effects are highly dependent upon total dose of radiation given, length of treatment, type of radiation delivered, and daily fractionated dose of radiation (Maher, 1996).

The Radiation Therapy Oncology Group (RTOG) has devised a grading system used to classify side effects for patients receiving RT. Grade 1 implies minor symptoms requiring no treatment or intervention, while grade 2 is designated by symptoms that impose no change in lifestyle or performance status and respond to simple outpatient therapy. Grade 3 is characterized by distressing symptoms affecting patient performance status and may require hospitalization for diagnosis or minor surgical and medical intervention. Grade 4 entails prolonged hospitalization or major medical or surgical intervention, and grade 5 is defined by fatal complications (Pilepich, Walz, & Baglan, 1987). The majority of patients receiving radiation therapy have grade 1 symptoms or no symptoms at all (Michalski et al., 2000; Pilepich, Walz, & Baglan, 1987). (See Tables 7.1 and 7.2 for the RTOG classification of acute and chronic urinary and bowel toxicities.)

FATIGUE: MANIFESTATIONS & ASSESSMENT

Most of the side effects related to radiation therapy are localized to the area being irradiated, however, fatigue is a symptom common to most patients receiving RT. It is estimated that approximately 65% to 100% of patients receiving RT experience fatigue (King, Nail, Kreamer, Strohl, & Johnson, 1985; Kubricht, 1984). Manifestations of fatigue include lack of energy, weakness, somnolence, impaired thought processes and mood disturbances. Because RT-related fatigue is a common side effect of treatment, patients need to be reminded that in no way does this represent worsening of the cancer. Fatigue has been documented as the most severe side effect of radiation, especially during the last week of treatment. The lowest incidence of fatigue was found in men receiving radiation to the pelvic area (i.e., men treated for prostate cancer) as compared to those receiving radiation to the chest (King, Nail, Kreamer, Strohl, & Johnson, 1985). Monga, Kerrigan, Thornby, and Monga (1999) investigated the degree of fatigue in men undergoing external beam RT for localized prostate cancer. They found that 25% of patients receiving RT for prostate cancer complained of fatigue at the completion of therapy.

Fatigue generally becomes evident around the middle of the treatment period and many patients characterize fatigue as having less energy. King and associates (1985) found fatigue to be worse and occur more frequently during the afternoon. It generally persists about one to three months after RT has been completed, but duration is dependent upon other concomitant factors and the individual patient. In fact, the incidence of fatigue one month after radiation in men receiving pelvic radiation was 58% and at three months the incidence of fatigue was 14%.

During the last decade, fatigue has been acknowledged as one of the most distressing and frustrating side effects associated with cancer and its treatment (Claus, Crow, & Hammond, 1996; McHale, 2000; Richardson, 1995). Nail and King (1987) defined fatigue as a human response to the experience of cancer and undergoing treatment for cancer. Aistars (1987) defines fatigue as a subjective feeling characterized by

TABLE 7.1 RTOG Acute Urinary and Pelvic Radiation Morbidity Scoring Criteria

Genitourinary

Grade	Symptom
Zero (0)	No change
One (1)	Frequency of urination or nocturia twice pretreatment habit Dysuria, urgency not requiring medication
Two (2)	Frequency of urination or nocturia which is less frequent than every hour Dysuria, urgency, bladder spasm requiring local anesthetic (e.g., Pyridium)
Three (3)	Frequency with urgency and nocturia hourly or more frequently Dysuria, pelvic pain, or bladder spasm requiring regular, frequent narcotic Gross hematuria with or without clot passage
Four (4)	Hematuria requiring transfusion Acute bladder obstruction not secondary to clot passage Ulceration or necrosis
Five (5)	Death related to radiation

Lower Gastrointestinal/Pelvic

Zero (0)	No change
One (1)	Increased frequency or change in quality of bowel habits not requiring medication Rectal discomfort not requiring analgesics
Two (2)	Diarrhea requiring parasympatholytic drugs (e.g., Lomotil) Mucous discharge not necessitating sanitary pads Rectal or abdominal pain requiring analgesics
Three (3)	Diarrhea requiring parenteral support Severe mucous or blood discharge necessitating sanitary pads Abdominal distention (flat plate radiograph demonstrates distended bowel loops)
Four (4)	Acute or subacute obstruction, fistula, or perforation GI bleeding requiring transfusion Abdominal pain or tenesmus requiring tube decompression or bowel diversion
Five (5)	Death

TABLE 7.2 RTOG/EORTC Late Radiation Morbidity Scoring Criteria for Bladder and Bowel

Bladder

Grade	Symptom
Zero (0)	None
One (1)	Slight epithelial atrophy Minor telangiectasia (microscopic hematuria)
Two (2)	Moderate frequency Generalized telangiectasia Intermittent macroscopic hematuria
Three (3)	Severe frequency and dysuria Severe generalized telangiectasia (often with petechiae) Frequent hematuria Reduction in bladder capacity (< 150 cc)
Four (4)	Necrosis Contracted bladder (capacity < 100 cc) Severe hemorrhagic cystitis
Five (5)	Death directly related to radiation late effects

Bowel

Grade	Symptom
Zero (0)	None
One (1)	Mild diarrhea Mild cramping Bowel movements 5 times daily Slight rectal discharge or bleeding
Two (2)	Moderate diarrhea and colic Bowel movements > 5 times daily Excessive rectal mucus or intermittent bleeding
Three (3)	Obstruction or bleeding, requiring surgery
Four (4)	Necrosis, perforation, or fistula
Five (5)	Death directly related to radiation late effects

generalized weariness, weakness, exhaustion, and lack of energy resulting from prolonged stress that is directly or indirectly attributable to the disease process. Piper's Integrated Fatigue model is the most frequently cited conceptual model of cancer-related fatigue. It includes perceptual, physiological, biochemical, and behavioral aspects of fatigue.

The exact phenomenon of fatigue and its relationship to radiation therapy is not well understood (Winningham et al., 1994). However, several theories have been postulated:

1. fatigue occurs to reserve energy for normal cellular repair (Hilderley, 1992);
2. radiation causes cellular destruction leading to by-product buildup, leading to fatigue (Hilderley, 1992);
3. the daily routine of radiation (i.e., five days per week) (Hilderley & Dow, 1991); and
4. its effect on erythrocytes leading to anemia (Ludwig & Fritz, 1998).

Many factors can contribute to the experience of fatigue. These may include concurrent or past chemotherapy, RT, anemia, infection, adverse effects of cancer itself, medications, medical or surgical treatments, inadequate rest, overexertion, poor nutrition, sleep disturbances, cancer progression or advanced disease, stress, anxiety, depression, uncontrolled diabetes, and presence of pain (Clark & Lacasse, 1998).

The assessment of fatigue is extremely important. Similar to pain, it is very subjective in nature. Many instruments have been developed to measure fatigue. Various instruments include the Multidimensional Fatigue Symptom Inventory (MFSI) developed by Stein, Martin, Hann, and Jacobsen (1998), the Brief Fatigue Inventory (BFI) developed by Mendoza and associates (1999), the Functional Assessment of Cancer Therapy—Fatigue Subscale (FACT-F) developed by Yellen, Cella, Webster, Blendowski, and Kaplan (1997), and the Piper Fatigue Scale developed by Piper and colleagues (1989). These instruments can be used to assist clinicians in quantifying fatigue and the impact it has on quality of life. Other contributing factors of fatigue must also be assessed in order to identify and implement interventions needed to minimize the impact of fatigue.

Fatigue: Management

The management of fatigue should be directed at decreasing fatigue or assisting the patient to adapt to fatigue. Most important, patients and family members need to be aware of impending fatigue and the various self-care activities to ease the symptom. Since RT-related fatigue typically occurs in the afternoon, patients may benefit from planning a nap or rest period. It is important to keep in mind that patients know their body better than anyone and should listen to what their body is telling them. When fatigue occurs, patients should take a nap or rest. When patients are feeling less tired or have more energy, there are no restrictions placed on their activities. Questions commonly asked by patients include: Will I be able to continue to keep working while undergoing radiation therapy? and Will I be able to drive myself to and from radiation? Most patients are able to drive themselves and even continue working. However, other factors may impact the ability of the patient to drive or ability to keep working. Therefore, a thorough assessment will help determine the activity plan that is appropriate for each individual patient.

Many patients keep a daily log or journal of their symptoms. This is helpful for anticipating symptoms, as well as planning ahead, scheduling activities and rest periods. Overexertion tends to exacerbate fatigue and should be avoided. It is important for the patient to identify energy-depleting activities, prioritize activities, reschedule events or activities around fatigue, delegate responsibilities to others, and rest when needed. Adequate nutrition is also essential in the management of fatigue. Small, frequent meals and snacks throughout the day, eating when appetite is the greatest, and drinking plenty of fluids will help maintain adequate nutritional balance and energy level. If nutritional disturbances or weight loss is evident, a referral to a dietitian may be warranted. Patients and their family members may also benefit from the NCI's publication *Eating Hints* and the ACS's publication *Nutrition for the Person with Cancer: A Guide for Patients & Families*.

Various studies have also examined exercise and its impact on level of fatigue. It is suggested that patients undergoing RT include exercise such as walking in their routine. Schwartz (2000) examined exercise and fatigue in women receiving chemotherapy for breast cancer and found that women who exercised had decreased fatigue and believed that exercise decreases the intensity of fatigue. No such studies have included men treated with RT for prostate cancer.

In addition to managing the symptoms of fatigue, contributing factors such as anemia, depression, anxiety, and sleep disturbances must be addressed. If a patient is anemic, management may include transfusion of packed red blood cells, vitamin or mineral supplements, or the administration of a colony-stimulating factor (i.e., Procrit®, Epogen®). Patients displaying symptoms of anxiety and depression may benefit from referral to an oncology social worker or psychiatric health care professional for evaluation and initiation of psychotherapy and anxiolytic or antidepressant therapy. Many cancer patients have sleep disturbances, characterized either by difficulty falling asleep or early awakening. Both can be predictors of anxiety and depression. Many appropriate sleeping aids can improve sleep problems. Ambien® (zolpidem tartrate) is a short-acting sleep aid, beneficial for those having difficulty falling asleep. Restoril® (temezapem) is longer acting and better for those experiencing early awakening. Sleep disturbances may also be caused by the presence of nocturia and pharmacologic intervention for urinary frequency may be needed. Therefore, it is important to complete a thorough patient history prior to initiating any interventions.

Cancer-related fatigue is a complex symptom, which is difficult to manage. Continued research is needed, especially for those men treated with external beam irradiation, brachytherapy, or combined modality for prostate carcinoma. As health care professionals, it is important to educate, support, and encourage patients to adapt and cope with fatigue.

ACUTE AND CHRONIC URINARY SYMPTOMS

Urinary Symptoms Associated with External Beam Radiation

The most common acute urinary symptoms associated with external radiation are related to cystitis, an inflammation and irritation of the bladder. These symptoms include frequency, nocturia, burning upon urination, dysuria, urgency, and to a lesser degree, urinary retention. Patients may also experience gross or microscopic hematuria. Urinary tract infections may also occur (Perez, Brady, & Chao, 1999). Dearnaley and colleagues (1999) compared side effects of conventional and conformal RT and found no significant difference in bladder symptoms. They found that approximately 50% of patients had grade 1 or 2 cystitis, but only 6% had dysuria.

Complication rates in the treatment of localized prostate cancer have decreased over the past 20 to 40 years as confirmed by the Prostate Cancer Clinical Guidelines Panel (Thompson et al., 1999). Even though the incidence of chronic effects has decreased and is relatively low, there can be bladder and rectal toxicities after RT. Hematuria, blood in the urine, can be a chronic problem associated with RT for prostate cancer. This is due to radiation damage to microvasculature of bladder lining. It occurs in about 3% to 8% of patients and may appear as gross or microscopic blood (Hanlon, Bruner, Peter, & Hanks, 2001; Dearnaley et al., 1999). It has been postulated that the risk of developing late bladder toxicities increased as the percentage of bladder receiving more than 65 Gy increased (Michalski et al., 2000).

Urinary incontinence (UI) can also be a side effect of RT; however, it is not nearly the problem that it is in men treated with radical prostatectomy. Chronic radiation changes include fibrosis, thinning of tissues, atrophy, and urethral strictures. UI usually occurs as a late or chronic effect of RT. Urinary incontinence has been estimated to occur in 1% to 2% of patients and slightly higher in those with a history of having a transurethral resection of prostate (TURP) (Perez, 1998). Incontinence can be classified into five types: 1) stress; 2) urge; 3) overflow; 4) mixed; and 5) total. The two types most commonly associated with RT are urge incontinence, which occurs when the bladder feels full and the desire to urinate is evident, and overflow incontinence, which is loss of urine caused by overfilling of bladder often associated with retention (Smith, 1999).

Urinary Symptoms Associated with Brachytherapy

Symptoms of radiation prostatitis usually start within the first to second week following the seed implantation and can persist for at least one to four months. However, Blasko and Wallner (1997) found that symptoms could last as long as 6 to 12 months, and even longer. They found that symptoms peaked at three to six weeks with Iodine-125, and two to three weeks with Palladium-103. Urinary symptoms following an implant include irritative and obstructive symptoms, such as urinary frequency, nocturia, dysuria, burning upon urination, weak stream, urgency, and urinary retention. Almost all patients develop some degree of dysuria and urinary frequency, both during the daytime and night. It has been reported that dysuria is the most common complaint of implantation, ranging from mild irritation to severe burning (Abel et al., 1999; Benoit, Naslund, & Cohen, 2000).

Acute urinary retention is another complication of implant therapy (Lee et al., 2000). The degree of severity is dependent on preexisting genitourinary symptoms, such as obstruction and benign prostatic hypertrophy. They also found that men who received three months of neoadjuvant hormone therapy with Pd-103, had more obstructive symptoms (Terk, Stock, & Stone, 1998). Another predictor of obstruction is the number of needles used to implant radioactive seeds (i.e., greater than 33) and the volume of the prostate (i.e., greater than 35 cm^3) (Lee et al., 2000). Occasionally radiation-induced edema or BPH can cause patients to display signs of severe urinary outlet obstruction in which they dribble or cannot urinate at all.

Late or chronic urinary complications occur 12 months or more after brachytherapy. Three percent to seven percent of patients may develop urinary outlet obstruction and retention that can persist throughout the life of the radioisotope. This may require a surgical intervention such as TURP (Benoit, Naslund, & Cohen, 2000; Blasko, Grimm, Ragde, & Schumacher, 1997; Ragde, Grado, Nadir, & Elgamal, 2000). Another complication is superficial urethral necrosis (SUN), which is the onset of irritative and obstructive symptoms 12 to 18 months after implantation. This is usually associated with previous transurethral resection of the prostate gland (TURP). There is an increased risk of SUN for patients who require TURP after implantation, which also increases risk of developing urinary incontinence (Blasko et al., 1997). Urinary incontinence may also occur as the result of having brachytherapy. It has been estimated that 5% to 13% of men develop urinary incontinence after brachytherapy (Benoit, Naslund, & Cohen, 2000; Ragde et al., 1997).

Assessment and Management of Urinary Symptoms

It is beneficial to assess urination symptoms before, during, and after RT. The American Urologic Association (AUA) Index is an instrument designed to measure symptoms of nocturia, urgency, weak urinary stream, feeling of incomplete emptying, frequency, inability to urinate, and decrease caliber and force of flow. Scores can range from zero to 35, with zero being the best score (Steele, Sullivan, Sleep, & Yalla, 2000). This type of instrument can be useful in assessing and predicting worsening symptoms once treatment begins and prevent or minimize them with the use of prophylactic medications. As mentioned earlier, the RTOG has developed a grading system for acute and chronic symptoms associated with RT.

It is recommended that patients undergoing daily external beam radiation see their radiation oncologist and nurse at least weekly, but more often if necessary. Patients receiving brachytherapy are assessed by telephone triage for any side effects related to the treatment and seen as needed. Assessment is based upon presence of acute urinary symptoms. If a patient complains of burning upon urination, it is important to rule out the presence of a urinary tract infection (UTI). A urinalysis and urine culture and sensitivity should be obtained. If no infection is present, the use of medications such as Pyridium® (phenazopyridine hydrochloride) and Pyridium Plus® are helpful in alleviating this symptom. The recommended dose is 200 mg BID to TID for at least 14 days. It is important to inform patients that Pyridium® changes the color of urine to bright orange and easily stains undergarments. Other medications that may aid in decreasing irritative urinary symptoms include Urispas® (flavoxate hydrochloride), which counteracts smooth muscle spasm of the urinary tract by relaxing the muscles. It helps to provide relief of dysuria, urgency, nocturia, frequency and incontinence due to cystitis. The recommended dose of Urispas® is 200 mg TID to QID.

If an infection is present, wait for the final sensitivity and use an appropriate antibiotic such as Cipro® (ciprofloxacin hydrochloride), Septra® (co-trimoxazole), or ampicillin sodium. The most common bacteria causing urinary tract infections is *E. coli*. Men with urinary tract infections (UTI) are considered to have complicated UTIs and should be treated for 10 to 14 days (Orenstein & Wong, 1999).

Frequency of urination and nocturia can be a hallmark sign of urinary retention, the incomplete evacuation of the bladder. If patients complain of frequent urination in small amounts, urinary retention must be considered. Various procedures can be performed to evaluate for post void residual volume such as straight catherization after voiding and use of uroflowmetry to evaluate contents of bladder. If urinary retention is present, the initiation of certain medications can be beneficial. Medications such as the alpha-adrenergic blockers, which include Cardura® (doxazosin mesylate), Hytrin® (terazosin hydrochloride), and the newest Flomax® (tamsulosin hydrochloride) may be used. Their mechanism of action is to decrease sympathetic tone on the vasculature and sympathetic nerves, resulting in better urine flow rate. Cardura® and Hytrin® are also used in the treatment of hypertension. The most common side effect associated with these drugs is postural hypotension, lightheadedness, and syncope. It is recommended that they be taken at bedtime. The recommended starting doses are 1 to 2 mg QHS and titrate cautiously to achieve expected response. Total dose should not exceed 10 mg QHS. Flomax® has a minimal effect on blood pressure, so no adjustments need to be made with concurrent antihypertensive regimen. The recommended dose is 0.4 mg QHS and can be increased to a maximum dose of 0.8 mg. Drug interactions have been reported with Flomax® and Tagamet® (cimetidine), Coumadin® (warfarin sodium), and the other alpha-adrenergic blockers. These medications are also used with patients that have benign prostatic hypertrophy (BPH), enlarged prostate not related to malignancy. It has been documented that about 50% of implant patients take these medications and about 20% will remain on the drug for at least two years after implantation (Blasko & Wallner, 1997). Medications such as antihistamines, cold and allergy medications containing pseudoephedrine sulfate, and oral decongestants are contraindicated in the presence of urinary retention, as they may exacerbate the condition.

It is oftentimes beneficial to use anti-inflammatory medications such as steroids, to aid in decreasing swelling and inflammation caused by the radiation. It is estimated that 33% of implant patients require the use of antispasmodics, such as Ditropan® (oxybutynin chloride), anti-inflammatory agents such as Medrol® (methylprednisolone), or nonsteroidal anti-inflammatory agents (NSAIDs) such as ibuprofen or naproxen, during this period. However, Zelefsky, Ginor, and Leibel (1999) compared the use of NSAIDs and alpha-adrenergic blockers and found that NSAIDs were less effective in treating urinary symptoms.

Management of severe urinary outlet obstruction, not relieved by pharmacological interventions, consists of the insertion of an indwelling urinary catheter or teaching the patient self-catherization. For urinary outlet obstruction and retention that persists beyond the life span of the radioisotope, treatment may include transurethral resection of the prostate (TURP) or cautery-knife incision of dorsal prostate and vesical neck.

Urinary incontinence, although a fairly infrequent side effect associated with RT, is a major concern for patients when it occurs. Assessment of urinary incontinence includes a thorough history, focusing on bladder functions such as episodes of incontinence, fluid intake, and number of absorbency pads used daily. The medical management of urinary incontinence includes the initiation of pelvic floor muscles, pharmacological interventions, and surgical interventions. Pelvic floor exercises, also known as Kegel exercises, assist in strengthening muscles and providing compensation of damaged external sphincter. The utilization of voiding schedules and biofeedback has been shown to be effective in the treatment of urinary incontinence (Harris, 1997). Medications which are helpful in minimizing urge incontinence include Pro-Banthine® (propantheline bromide), Bentyl® (dicyclomine hydrochloride), Ditropan® (oxybutynin chloride), and Tofranil® (imipramine hydrochloride), which act as anticholinergics or smooth muscle relaxants. The most recent FDA-approved drug for urge incontinence is Detrol® (tolterodine tartrate), which is a muscarinic receptor antagonist. It assists in increasing residual urine, thereby decreasing urge incontinence.

Surgical interventions are generally utilized in the radical prostatectomy patients. The management of urinary incontinence is not just medical, in that the psychosocial aspects need to be addressed as well. Incontinence brings about feelings of embarrassment, social isolation, anger, and issues of decreased quality of life (Harris, 1997). The attendance in a prostate cancer support group or individual psychotherapy may be helpful in dealing with these issues.

ACUTE AND CHRONIC RECTAL SYMPTOMS

Rectal Symptoms Associated with External Beam Radiation

Rectal symptoms are also common in men receiving external beam RT for prostate cancer. This occurs as a result of radiation to local rectal tissue that is in close proximity to the prostate gland. In the acute period, normal cells become inflamed and edematous. Common side effects include frequent bowel movements with change in fecal consistency, increased flatulence, tenesmus, proctitis and hemorrhoidal irritation. Diarrhea is less common in men receiving 3DCRT as compared to those receiving conventional method therapy (Hanlon et al., 2001). Tenesmus is the persistent feeling of incomplete evacuation of stool from the rectum. Men often complain of rectal pressure with pelvic irradiation. Another side effect of pelvic radiation is rectal urgency with or without incontinence. This is caused by dysfunction of internal and external anal sphincters. Yeoh and colleagues (1998) reported that 23% of men receiving external RT to the pelvis, with total dose ranging from 55 to 64 Gy, experienced fecal incontinence for at least four to six weeks after treatment.

Another side effect is proctitis, which is inflammation of the rectal mucosa and commonly occurs with patients receiving pelvic radiation. It is manifested by mucus-like, bloody and painful defecation. Edema and fibrosis of the arterioles of colonic mucosa result in radiation proctitis. As the fibrosis enhances, the mucosa becomes friable and bleeding occurs. The gastroenterology literature has reported an increased risk of developing proctitis with the presence of comorbid vascular conditions such as diabetes, hypertension, and chronic inflammatory bowel diseases (Gelblum & Potters, 2000). Dearnaley and others (1999) found the most common bowel side effect was proctitis, which usually presented as rectal bleeding. They reported grade 1 or higher toxicities occurred in 56% of the conventional group as compared to 37% in the conformal therapy group.

Hemorrhoidal or perineal irritation is also common and is manifested by erythema and dry desquamation. Constipation has also been documented with radiation to the pelvis. Decreased rectosigmoid motility and spasms commonly cause this (Counter, Froese, & Hart, 1999; Earnest, 1991).

Acute bladder and bowel toxicities in the preliminary report of 3DOG/RTOG 94-06 were found to be very favorable. This cooperative study looked at acute bladder and bowel toxicities utilizing 3DCRT dose escalations, ranging from 68.4 to 73.8 Gy. They found acute bladder and bowel tolerance to be favorable, with 53% to 62% of patients having experienced grade 1 or no toxicities at all. The incidence of grade 2 toxicities ranged from 18% to 31% whereas the incidence of grade 3 toxicities was 0% to 3% (Michalski et al., 2000).

Chronic proctitis and rectal bleeding are the most common late sequelae of high dose 3DCRT as researched by Teshima, Hanks, Hanlon, Peter, and Schultheiss (1997) at Fox Chase Cancer Center. Chronic proctitis can occur if cells become fibrotic and ischemia develops (Earnest, 1991). Teshima and others (1997) have reported that rectal bleeding can develop 6 to 12 months after treatment and last for the duration of three months. It is recommended that appropriate shielding of the rectal mucosa take place in order to limit radiation dose to < 72 Gy and avoid chronic rectal complications. It has been found that 90% of gastrointestinal complications occur by two and a half years post-treatment (Benoit, Naslund, & Cohen, 2000).

Chronic bladder and bowel toxicities were found to be minimal in the preliminary results of 3DOG/RTOG 94-06 study. Approximately 81% to 85% of patients had either none or grade 1 toxicity, while 2% to 10% of patients experienced grade 2 symptoms. Only one patient suffered a grade 3 bladder complication and no grade 4 or 5 toxicities were reported. Most late effects occurred within 12 to 18 months of treatment (Michalski et al., 2000).

Rectal Symptoms Associated with Prostate Brachytherapy

Rectal symptoms associated with brachytherapy are minimal. These symptoms include change in bowel pattern, proctitis, tenesmus, hemorrhoidal irritation, and rectal bleeding. Patients commonly experience more frequent bowel movements after implant therapy (Blasko et al., 1997). It has been investigated that there is no correlation between increasing rectal toxicity and the use of combined treatment modality with external bean irradiation and seed implantation (Gelbaum & Potters, 2000; Merrick et al., 2000).

Chronic rectal symptoms related to implant therapy are also minimal. Proctitis was an infrequent side effect and occurred in about 3% of patients. The most feared complication after brachytherapy is the development of a prostatic-rectal fistula and occurs in approximately 0.3% of patients (Blasko et al., 1997; Benoit, Naslund, & Cohen, 2000).

Assessment and Management of Rectal Symptoms

Rectal symptoms are more problematic in the patient receiving external beam irradiation as compared to implant patients. Assessment of normal bowel pattern prior to radiation is important. These factors include number of bowel movements per day, consistency and color of stool. Radiation to the prostate region generally causes irritation and inflammation of rectum, leading to more frequent bowel movements, changes in consistency, feeling of incomplete evacuation, proctitis and hemorrhoidal irritation. Interventions helpful in minimizing symptoms of frequent bowel movements or diarrhea include Imodium-AD® (loperamide hydrochloride), Lomotil® (diphenoxylate hydrochloride & atropine sulfate), and bulk-forming laxative such as Metamucil® (psyllium). Metamucil® may also be effective in relieving symptoms of constipation. The initiation of a low residue diet may also be beneficial in decreasing number of bowel movements and referral to dietitian may also be helpful.

The treatment of tenesmus is the administration of steroid-based enemas containing hydrocortisone or enemas containing 5-aminosalicylic acid (5-ASA) like Rowasa®, and the use of muscle relaxants or sedatives for severe tenesmus. Another option for severe tenesmus is Azulfidine® (oral sulfasalazine), which is also used in the management of Crohn's disease and ulcerative colitis. Proctitis is treated with the use of hydrocortisone enemas such as Proctofoam®, Cortifoam® and the use of rectal suppositories containing bismuth, zinc oxide, or cortisone. They include Anusol®, Anusol HC®, Rowasa®, and Wyanoids®. In the case of severe rectal bleeding or proctitis, the use of laser therapy or hyperbaric oxygen has been beneficial.

Hemorrhoidal irritation or skin reaction can occur and be managed with the use of Sitz baths and application of ointments such as Aquaphor®. Often times, Aquaphor® can be combined with Xylocaine 5% ointment®, to enhance comfort.

SEXUAL DYSFUNCTION IN THE PATIENT WITH PROSTATE CANCER

Sexual dysfunction in the prostate cancer population receiving radiation therapy occurs in 14% to 50% of patients and is dependent upon age and radiation technique. More qualitative assessment is needed to further evaluate this quality of life issue (Perez, Brady, & Chao, 1999). Peschel (1997) has estimated that 48% to 59% of patients receiving external beam irradiation for prostate cancer have some sexual potency. Other researchers have found that the difference between conventional therapy and 3DCRT in terms of sexual dysfunction is similar (Roach, Chinn, Holland, & Clark, 1996; Mantz et al., 1997). For a complete discussion of the assessment and management of sexual dysfunction in the prostate cancer patient, see chapter 10.

FUTURE DIRECTIONS

With the advances in radiation oncology in the prostate cancer arena, the role of the nurse will become increasingly more important and essential. As a primarily outpatient treatment, the acuity of patients has increased along with the complexity of care provided to patients. New directions in the field of radiation oncology in the treatment of prostate cancer include intense modulated radiation therapy (IMRT), high dose rate (HDR) brachytherapy, and stereotactic radiosurgery. The role of the oncology nurse continues to expand with respect to the physical and psychosocial needs of the patient and their family. However, more research and clinical studies are needed that will examine quality of life issues such as fatigue, sexual dysfunction and psychosocial issues.

SUMMARY

The role of the nurse caring for the patient with prostate cancer is complex and multifaceted and certainly challenging in nature. Nursing care must be focused on the physical limitations of the disease and on managing side effects of treatment in order to enhance quality of life. The mind and body connection cannot be overlooked, and the assessment and management of psychosocial issues must be met. Cancer is a family disease, and although the family is not effected physically, the magnitude of emotions is great. Throughout the trajectory of prostate cancer, all these issues need to be assessed and managed to provide quality of care to patients with prostate cancer.

8
Hormone Therapy

Dorothy A. Calabrese

Prior to the use of prostate specific antigen (PSA) as a screening tool, patients with prostate cancer were usually diagnosed with locally advanced or metastatic prostate cancer. The widespread use of the PSA blood test has changed the profile of patients currently diagnosed with prostate cancer. Many patients are now diagnosed with a localized cancer, one that is at a potentially curable stage (Haas & Resnick, 2000; Seay et al., 1997). Despite this progress in screening men, there are men each year who at the initial urologic evaluation are still diagnosed with metastatic prostate cancer. In addition, metastatic disease will develop later in a percentage of men who have had definitive treatment. For these patients, hormone therapy is the current treatment of choice.

Patients who are diagnosed with extracapsular extension of the cancer outside the prostate and men who are diagnosed with cancer that has spread to other parts of the body will most likely not be cured of their cancer. In 2001, approximately 31,500 men will die from prostate cancer, and the incidence and mortality rates are considerably higher among African American men when compared to Caucasians, Asians, and Native Americans (Smith et al., 2001). The focus of care for these patients is how to best manage the prostate cancer without significant treatment side effects that would affect their quality of life (QOL).

Just as this change toward earlier stage at diagnosis has occurred, the use of hormone therapy to treat patients with prostate cancer has changed. Several years ago, when a patient asked how long he would be on hormone medication, the answer would be "for the rest of your life." The answer to that question today isn't as clear cut as it once was. Currently the answer depends upon the specifics of why the patient is receiving the hormone medication, as well as developing knowledge about prostate cancer and the use of hormone therapy as treatment.

Hormone treatment is the gold standard for the treatment of metastatic prostate cancer, and it has also become the gold standard for treatment for recurrent disease (Fitch et al., 2000). The goal of treatment is palliation and prolonging survival in patients with advanced prostate cancer. Even though androgen ablation has been used for many years, controversies related to initiation of therapy, the use of intermittent hormone therapy, preferable forms of androgen therapy, and the role of complete androgen blockade remain (Klotz, 2000; Moul, 1998). This chapter will discuss the use of hormone therapy for the treatment of metastatic prostate cancer. The physiological influence of hormones on prostate cancer growth as well as the manipulation of these hormones to control the disease will be specifically addressed. The various types of hormone therapy and the nursing care necessary for the administration of the therapy, albeit scant, will be reviewed. The chapter will conclude with a discussion of chemotherapy to treat prostate cancer—the nursing implications of hormone and chemotherapy.

EFFECT OF HORMONES ON PROSTATE TISSUE GROWTH

The effect of hormone therapy in the treatment of prostate cancer was first described by Huggins, Stevens, and Hodges in the 1940s. Their work identified the importance of androgens in prostate cancer and described the effect of castration on advanced prostate cancer (Huggins et al., 1941; Daw & Peereboom, 2000). These observations are the basis for learning how hormone therapy could be used to treat prostate cancer.

Andogens regulate the growth of prostate tissue. Androgen effects the prostate cells when the hypothalamus secretes luteinizing hormone-releasing hormone (LHRH), which is then carried to the pituitary. The presence of LHRH stimulates the release of Luteinizing hormone (LH) by the pituitary. LH stimulates cells in the testicles, leading to the production of testosterone. Testosterone is converted in the prostate by the action of 5 alpha reductase to dihydrotestosterone (DHT). DHT is the most metabolically active androgen in the regulation of prostate growth, stimulating protein synthesis and inhibiting prostate cell death. In addition the adrenal glands produce a small amount (5% to 10%) of testosterone that is circulated throughout the body. The production of the sex steroids delta-4-androstenedione, dihydroepiandrosterone (DHEA) and DHEA sulfate (DHEA-S) produced by the adrenal glands are also converted to DHT by enzymes found in the prostate (Daw & Peereboom, 2000).

USE OF HORMONE MANIPULATION

The different methods of hormone therapy options are based on disruption of the hypothalamic-pituitary-gonadal axis by medical or surgical means. There are four major methods of hormone therapy: bilateral orchiectomy or removal of the testicles, the primary androgen-producing organs; decreasing of production of luteinizing hormone (LH) by the use of estrogen or luteinizing hormone releasing hormone (LHRH) agonists; inhibition of androgen action at the target organs by antiandrogen medication; or combined androgen blockade (CAB) (Daw & Peereboom, 2000). The use of any of these methods depends not only upon the stage of the cancer, but also on the preference of the patient and the physician.

There are several different periods during the prostate cancer disease trajectory when hormone therapy is appropriate. While most men currently present with localized disease at the time of diagnosis, some patients present with extensive metastatic prostate cancer. Typical complaints or symptoms that prompt men to seek medical attention may include pain, fatigue, decreased mobility, constipation, scrotal edema, or urinary retention (Fitch et al., 2000). For these patients, the focus of hormone therapy goes beyond symptom control to QOL issues related to disease progression and survival. Eighty percent of men experiencing symptoms from prostate cancer will respond to hormone therapy with both objective responses (e.g., decrease in tumor size, lower PSA, reduced urinary obstructive symptoms, reduced bone pain) and subjective responses (e.g., improved appetite or sense of well-being) (Stempkowski, 2000).

Hormone therapy can also be used neoadjuvantly, that is, prior to definitive treatment for localized prostate cancer (e.g., before radiation therapy) to improve treatment outcomes. It can also be used after therapy to prolong the effects of local therapy (Stempkowski, 2000; Ziada et al., 2000). For example, significant numbers of prostate cancer patients will show recurrence following surgery or radiation therapy. Approximately 50% of men may be understaged clinically and later found to have tumors that extend beyond the prostate capsule at the time of surgery (Moul, 1998; Stempkowski, 2000). Patients who experience recurrence of prostate cancer based on a rising PSA often have a very different prognosis than a person diagnosed with metastatic prostate cancer. However, hormone therapy is also effective when used during both periods, along the prostate cancer trajectory (Klotz, 2000).

The natural history of progression of prostate cancer is unknown. Decisions about initiating hormone treatment need to take into account the need to stop the spread of the disease and the side effects of the treatment. Besides the side effects of the therapy, the men may face issues related to sexual function, anger, fear of dying, and fear of pain.

TYPES OF HORMONE THERAPY

The goal of hormone therapy is to stop the growth and spread of prostate cancer cells. This is accomplished by stopping the production of testosterone in the testicles, thus keeping the prostate cancer cells from spreading. There are several ways to accomplish this. Early options included taking oral estrogen or having a bilateral orchiectomy. Diethylstilbestrol (DES) has been used to suppress the production of testosterone; however, it is rarely used today due to the associated untoward cardiovascular side effects (Moul, 1998).

Current hormonal manipulation methods involve either medical castration through the use of LHRH agonists or surgical castration (i.e., bilateral orchiectomy). Since these methods have the same effect, the side effects are similar. These effects include hot flashes, decreased libido, impotence, and fatigue. Weight redistribution and muscle atrophy may also occur. A late effect can be osteoporosis due to the hormonal influence on bone's ability to compete for circulating calcium.

Surgical castration is the gold standard for removal of circulating testosterone. Within several hours following surgery, there is approximately a 95% reduction of circulating testosterone (Daw & Peereboom, 2000). There are several advantages to bilateral orchiectomy. In addition to the rapid reduction of the testosterone level, bilateral orchiectomy avoids a major testosterone surge common with LHRH agonists. Bilateral orchiectomy is a method that ensures patient compliance, since it is a one time outpatient procedure with minimal risks. The cost is low; even though there are surgical, anesthesia, and operating room costs. Since the result is a lifetime deprivation of testosterone, there is a major cost saving in comparison to use of LHRH agonists. The major disadvantage is that many men find the thought of having their testicles removed psychologically unpalatable, feeling that this affects their body image and perception of masculinity. Since it is a permanent procedure, the irreversibility may be a disadvantage if there are significant side effects. Bilateral orchiectomy also prevents patients from participating in any treatment methods that may be developed in the future.

Medical castration involves the use of the LHRH® agonist Lupron® (leuprolide) or Zoladex® (goserelin) to decrease the production of testosterone to castrate levels (< 20 ng/ml). The LHRH agonist eliminates the pulsatile LHRH stimulation by inhibiting the LH secretion from the pituitary. The continuous LHRH stimulation leads to a desensitization of the pituitary gland resulting in inhibition of LH production. The first dose of an LHRH agonist increases the testosterone level, called a "tumor flare," due to the increased LH production induced by the LHRH agonist. This increase in testosterone level lasts approximately five to eight days.

Desensitization of the pituitary gland occurs, and testosterone levels fall (Stempkowski, 2000). The testosterone level then falls to castrate levels. This flare phenomena is particularly important in patients with spinal cord metastasis or urinary obstruction, since the effects of the symptoms can become worse during this phase. This surge of testosterone can be eliminated by administration of an antiandrogen agent, such as Flutamide® (eulixin), Casodex® (bicalutamide), and Nilandrone® (nilutamide) for five to seven days prior to beginning the LHRH agonist. The antiandrogen blocks the use of testosterone at the androgen receptor sites.

The frequency of administration and dosage of the LHRH agonist depends upon the medication. Lupron® is administered intramuscularly, while Zoladex® is administered subcutaneously. Lupron® depot 22.5 mg is administered every 12 weeks or 30 mg is given every 16 weeks. Zoladex® 10.8 mg is administered every 12 weeks. The longer acting depot formulations are more convenient for patients, but they are costly. Their cost is usually covered by Medicare and most other insurance carriers.

The main side effects of the LHRH agonists are the same as those listed for bilateral orchiectomy (e.g., hot flashes, decreased libido, impotence, muscle wasting, fatigue). Patients also occasionally experience discomfort at the injection site. This latter effect is self-limiting and resolves spontaneously.

The choice between LHRH agonists versus bilateral orchiectomy is a very individual one. While there has been no difference shown between bilateral orchiectomy and use of LHRH agonists in keeping the prostate cancer cells from spreading, patients in the United States favor the use of LHRH agonists (Moul, 1998).

ANTIANDROGEN MEDICATIONS

Antiandrogen medications are nonsteroidal compounds that directly bind to the androgen receptor site without altering the peripheral testosterone level (Stempkowski, 2000). They can be used alone, called monotherapy. However, they are often used in combination with the LHRH agonists, complete androgen blockade or CAB. There are three antiandrogen medications presently available: Flutamide® (eulixin), Casodex® (bicalutamide), and Nilandrone® (nilutamide). Flutamide® is the oldest of these medications; the dosage is 250 mg (two tablets) every eight hours. Casodex's® dosage is one 50-mg tablet daily. The Nilandrone® dosage is also 50 mg per day.

The main side effects of the antiandrogen medications are breast tenderness, gynecomastia, hot flashes, and anemia. Liver dysfunction associated with elevated liver function enzymes has been reported with all three of the antiandrogen medications, but the incidence has been low, and discontinuing the medication usually results in liver enzymes returning to normal limits (Stempkowski, 2000). Diarrhea has also been reported by patients taking Flutamide®; resolution usually results when the patient's dosage is adjusted to one capsule every eight hours.

Patients taking Nilandrone® reported delayed adaptation to darkness (Newton & Kosier, 1998). In one study light-dark adaptation problems were reported by 12 of 18 patients (67%) (Dole & Holdsworth, 1997) and in another study, only 5 of 225 patients experienced "troublesome" transient visual disturbances (Janknegt et al., 1993). Despite the variance in experiencing this side effect, it is important that patients are made aware of this effect prior to starting the medication. Another possible side effect with Nilandrone is a reversible interstitial lung disease. The condition usually begins within three months of starting the medication, and resolves when the medication is stopped (Stempkowski, 2000). Symptoms include progressive exertional dyspnea, cough, chest pain, and fever.

Antiandrogen medications are not covered by Medicare. Prescription plans usually cover the cost of the medication. For patients who do not have a prescription plan, the antiandrogen medications are costly. While costs vary geographically, they also may vary from pharmacy to pharmacy in the same city. A month's supply of the medication costs approximately $300. The pharmaceutical companies that produce these medications typically have financial assistance programs to help patients obtain the medications if cost is a factor.

Interest in use of the antiandrogen medications as monotherapy is increasing. In an analysis of two studies in which 480 men in Denmark with stage T3/4 prostate cancer were randomized to either 150 mg of Casodex or medical or surgical castration, there was statistically no significant difference between the two groups in overall survival after 6.3 years (Iverson et al., 2000). The main benefits to monotherapy are to preserve sexual function and prevent the side effects related to suppression of testosterone (Boccardo, 2000).

In addition to the nonsteroidal antiandrogens, there are steroidal antiandrogen medications that inhibit the LH secretion from the pituitary and block testosterone at the receptor level. Cyproterone acetate (CPA) is the medication of this class that has been studied the most. While it is used in Europe and Canada, it is not approved for use in the United States. Megace® (megestrol acetate) is a medication of this class that has been used in the United States.

COMPLETE ANDROGEN BLOCKADE

Much has been written about the use of complete or total androgen blockade (CAB). The rationale is to block the production of testosterone by the use of medical or surgical castration and block its androgen receptor use by adding an antiandrogen medication to the regime. The goal is total androgen suppression. The clinical benefits continue to be debated. The ultimate question is whether survival benefits outweigh the additional cost and side effects. Studies continue to show conflicting results on these questions. Some studies show a symptomatic benefit to CAB as well as a survival benefit. Other studies have not confirmed the survival benefit but do show a benefit for symptom control. A study by Crawford and associates (1989) showed that patients with metastatic prostate cancer stratified with regard to extent of disease, performance status, and with limited disease and treated with CAB, survived longer than patients treated by castration. However, another study by Crawford compared the use of an antiandrogen with and without an orchiectomy, did not demonstrate a survival difference between the two arms (Crawford et al., 1997). Due to the wide disparities in trial design, a meta-analysis of these data has not been helpful in answering the questions regarding survival. Current data analysis supports the use of CAB. The data show that antiandrogen monotherapy alone is inferior to CAB and surgical or medical castration alone is also inferior or at best equal to combination therapies (Ziada et al., 2000).

Complete androgen blockade may be accomplished in several ways. One commonly used method employs the combination of an LHRH agonist with the use of an antiandrogen. Bilateral orchiectomy plus an antiandrogen is another method. Either method should result in decreased production and use of testosterone in the prostate cancer patient. The patient on CAB can experience the side effects from both the LHRH agonist and the antiandrogen: hot flashes, fatigue, breast tenderness, decreased libido, impotence, muscle wasting, and gynecomastia.

INTERMITTENT HORMONE THERAPY

Intermittent hormone therapy is the use of an LHRH agonist, with or without an antiandrogen, on an intermittent basis. When the patient's PSA level approaches zero, the hormone medication is stopped. The PSA levels are followed at regular predetermined intervals. When the PSA rises to a predetermined level, often 10 ng/ml, the hormone treatment is resumed. The interest in this method of treatment for prostate cancer has been driven mostly by patients, and studies on animals and in vitro cell-lines suggest that intermittent hormone therapy is beneficial. However, long-term data on human studies for safety and efficacy are not yet available (Moul, 1998; Daw & Peereboom, 2000). Since many of the side effects from hormone treatment are decreased during the time off hormone therapy, patients often anecdotally describe an improved sense of well-being while off the hormone medication.

RED FLAG SYMPTOMS

The patient with prostate cancer can experience many problems during his course of treatment. Although this is not unique for any cancer patient, there are several symptoms in men receiving hormonal therapy for prostate cancer that are important for the patient to identify and report to the health care professional before the symptoms result in a medical emergency.

Pain is a symptom that often occurs in patients with cancer, and the patient with prostate cancer is no exception. If a patient has metastatic disease to the spine, and he experiences an increase in back pain with a concurrent change in bowel and/or bladder symptoms (incontinence or urinary retention, diarrhea or constipation), spinal cord compression must always be considered. This is a medical emergency and one in which the patient needs to be evaluated immediately. Initiating intravenous steroids and radiation therapy to the spine may keep the patient from a spinal cord compression and possible paralysis.

Another area of concern is changing urinary symptoms. Most men with prostate cancer experience a variety of urinary symptoms: dysuria, urgency, frequency, straining to start their stream. The nurse and patient both need to be alert to a change or worsening of symptoms. If a patient is not able to fully empty the bladder, he is at risk for infection as well as for kidney damage due to urine backing up into the kidney and damaging nephrons. How to treat the inability to empty the bladder will depend upon the specifics of the situation and can include resection of prostate tissue, placement of a Foley catheter, intermittent self-catheterization, or placement of nephrostomy tubes. Early intervention can prevent a worsening of a problem that can result in long-term sequelae as well as a great deal of discomfort for the patient.

HORMONE REFRACTORY PROSTATE CANCER

Prostate cancer typically responds to hormone therapy. If the man is experiencing symptoms related to the prostate cancer, they lessen. The hormone therapy keeps the prostate cancer from spreading. Historically, the median response time to androgen ablation is cited at 12 to 16 months (Stempkowski, 2000). Patients on CAB typically experience progressive disease within 12 to 16 months after starting treatment (Daw & Peereboom,

2000). That time frame will vary and is dependant upon the tumor burden and the aggressiveness of the tumor. However, inevitably, the prostate cancer cells will become androgen-independent, that is, they will grow and spread and will not need testosterone as fuel. This androgen-independence is thought to be due to the heterogeneity of the prostate tumor, and survival following the failure of hormone therapy is 9 to 18 months (Daw & Peereboom, 2000).

The goals at this stage of the prostate cancer trajectory are to delay and prevent complications, shrink the cancer, lower the PSA, improve symptoms, and extend the patient's lifespan. The manner in which this is best accomplished is an ongoing challenge to those working with the prostate cancer patient population.

When a patient is on hormone therapy and the PSA begins to rise, there are several things that can and should be done. It is important to ensure that the testosterone level is at a castrate level (< 20 ng/ml). If the patient is on an LHRH agonist, he should continue on it, since this is keeping much of the prostate cancer under control. If the patient is not on an antiandrogen, it is reasonable to begin an antiandrogen to see what effect this will have on the PSA level. If the patient is on an antiandrogen, the medication should be stopped (antiandrogen withdrawal syndrome). This is the first step for men who have demonstrated a rise in PSA despite androgen ablation.

The patient most likely to benefit from the antiandrogen withdrawal syndrome is the one who has been on CAB for more than a year. Stopping the antiandrogen causes a decrease in the PSA level and an improvement in clinical symptoms (Stempkowski, 2000). When Flutamide is the antiandrogen stopped, the withdrawal effect is seen quickly due to its short half life (5.2 hours). For patients taking Casodex®, the PSA can continue rising for approximately seven weeks before it begins to decline (again due to the long half-life of one week) (Stempkowski, 2000).

When the PSA again begins to rise, secondary hormones (or endocrine) therapy can be instituted. There are a variety of methods used to introduce secondary hormone therapy with some success. The use of corticosteroids to suppress the pituitary production of corticotropin (and indirectly decrease the production of adrenal androgens) shows a 20% to 25% response rate. Medications used include oral prednisone, dexamethasone, and hydrocortisone. Ketoconazole®, an antifungal, inhibits both testicular and adrenal androgen production. A dosage of 200 mg to 400 mg three times per day has demonstrated a response rate of 20% to 30%. Adding hydrocortisone to Ketoconazole has a 50% response rate that lasts three to four months (Stempkowski, 2000). The side effects include nausea, vomiting, skin rash, nail changes, edema, hepatotoxicity, and gynecomastia.

Aminogultethimide suppresses adrenal androgen production. Administered with hydrocortisone, it has a response rate of 0% to 40%. The side effects include lethargy, nausea, skin rashes, peripheral edema, hypothyroidism, and abnormal liver enzymes.

Estrogen suppresses the pituitary gonadotropin leading to decreased testosterone secretion. DES 1 mg to 3 mg is used daily, and it has a response rate of 15% to 20%. Side effects include thromboembolic events, nausea, vomiting, fluid retention, gynecomastia, and changes in liver enzymes.

Progestins inhibit tumor growth. Medroxyprogesterone acetate is used primarily to reduce bone pain. Side effects include peripheral edema and a risk for cardiovascular events. Megace® (megestrol acetate) has minimal effect in hormone refractory disease, but is used to help in hot flashes symptom relief.

The secondary hormone therapies produce minimal benefit in patients with hormone refractory disease. Response rates, if they occur, are usually of short duration. Patients at this point in time may want to consider participation in a clinical trial.

CHEMOTHERAPY

Historically, patients with prostate cancer have had poor response to single-agent chemotherapy (Held-Warmkessel, 2000; Kamradt & Pienta, 2000). Measurement of response to the chemotherapy treatment had been an ongoing issue in treating these patients. Measurement of soft tissue disease and bone metastasis can be difficult and unreliable. This made the measurement of response to chemotherapy difficult. Often if the patient responded to the treatment, he was declared "clinically stable" which can mean one of several different things. There could objectively be a reduction in tumor size; there could be an improvement in well being; or there could be a decrease in the marker being measured (Kamradt & Pienta, 2000). When PSA became a commonly used tumor marker, it helped to usher in a new era in treating hormone-resistant prostate cancer. This readily available blood test allowed a broader patient population to be included in clinical trials. An example is patients with bone metastases and an elevated PSA. The clinical trials that use a decrease in PSA as a measure of tumor response have resulted in an increased response rate. The response rate in these "first" generation regimes is approximately 50%. The National Comprehensive Cancer Network (NCCN) suggests a trial of chemotherapy as a treatment option for advanced disease (Kamradt & Pienta, 2000).

A patient's decision to participate in a clinical trial depends upon several factors: the extent of the tumor, the rate of the tumor growth, the presence and severity of his symptoms, his general medical condition, and the willingness to tolerate the side effects of chemotherapy (Held-Warmkessel, 2000). The uncertain benefits as well as an uncertain future makes participation in a clinical trial a very difficult decision. The patient needs to decide when to begin treatment, since the person often feels well when he reaches this crossroad. Waiting too long may make a person ineligible to participate in the trial, since he may not meet the eligibility requirements. Often a man is unwilling to participate in a program that will make him feel unwell due to side effects without a guarantee of a positive benefit for him.

There are several chemotherapy regimes currently reported in the literature that are showing favorable outcomes. For example, Ketoconazole®, an antifungal medication (1,200 mg per day) combined with Doxorubicin (20 mg/m^2 over 24 hours) is being studied in a Phase II trial. In a trial to test the effectiveness of Ketoconazole® and Doxorubicin, 39 patients who had progressive prostate cancer following initial hormone therapy were treated on this protocol. Approximately 55% of patients had a PSA decline of greater than 50% (a significant variable in predicting survival) and 58% had partial response of measurable disease. (Kamradt & Pienta, 2000).

While Vinblastine® has shown minimal response as a single agent to treat prostate cancer, its use in combination with Estramustine® has demonstrated synergistic cytotoxicity. The therapy has been well tolerated at dosages for Vinblastine® of 4 mg/m^2 weekly and for Estramustine® at 10 mg/kg daily for six weeks followed by a two-week rest period. Kamradt and Pienta found that response rates varied from 10% to 40% in bidimensional measurement of disease; PSA declines of more than 50% occurred in 54% to 61% of the patients.

Etoposide® and Estramustine® are cytotoxic agents that have been used in combination to treat prostate cancer. These drugs are given orally. Estramustine's® dosage is 15 mg/kg/day, and the dosage for Etoposide® is 50 mg/m^2/day. The medications are given for a three-week period followed by a one-week rest period. Approximately 50% of patients had objective responses, and a PSA decline of more than 50% occurred in 55% of patients on the study (Kamradt & Pienta, 2000).

Mitoxanthrone® (12 mg/m^2 every 21 days) and prednisone (10 mg/day) has been used in several different clinical trials. The complete response rate reported is 36%, while 44% of the patients experienced a partial response rate. In addition there was a reduction in use of analgesia. These results were replicated in a larger study, and the duration of the response was 43 weeks (Kamradt & Pienta, 2000).

The combination of Paclitaxel® (120 mg/m^2 by 96-hour continuous infusion every 21 days) and Estramustine® (600 mg/m^2/day) has demonstrated a synergistic cytotoxic effect. Approximately 44% of patients had objective response, and a PSA decline of more than 50% occurred in 53% of patients. The median duration of response was 37 weeks (Kamradt & Pienta, 2000).

This is an exciting time in prostate cancer research. Clinical trials are ongoing with a variety of chemotherapy agents. The goal of these trials is to identify the best regimes for the treatment of hormone resistant prostate cancer. Several new chemotherapy regimes have shown promise and will likely provide the basis of future clinical trials. The trials include: Paclitaxel®, Estramustine®, and Etoposide®; Docetaxel® and Estramustine®; and chemohormonal therapy with Doxorubicin®, Ketoconazole®, Vinblastine®, and Estramustine® (Kamradt & Pienta, 2000). These are just several of the clinical trials that are in progress to help find additional and better ways to treat androgen independent prostate cancer patients.

Besides the chemotherapy protocols that are evolving, other methods of therapy are being investigated. These include antiangiogenesis therapy, a method to prevent neovascularization and subsequent growth of prostate cancer; differentiation therapy, a method to arrest the growth of prostate cancer by using metabolites of protein to induce apoptosis; gene therapy; and antimetastatic therapy, a method that uses anti-invasion therapy and antiadhesion agents (Kamradt & Pienta, 2000).

NURSING IMPLICATIONS

Nurses play a key role in patient education and side effect management in patients on hormone therapy. Patients often hesitate to discuss side effects of treatment, fears, and/or anxieties with their physicians because of the doctors' busy schedule. Yet with a little encouragement, the nurse is often able to assess the issues that are paramount to the patient.

The nurse's role begins when a patient, along with his wife or significant other, is considering treatment options. The person is given a great deal of information in a short time period, and he will probably not absorb the majority of it at that time. Providing written information on hormone therapy, side effects, and the management of the side effects will provide the patient with necessary information to make an informed decision about his treatment. For men with metastatic prostate cancer, the treatment options are limited, but there are options for the patient to consider (e.g., medical versus surgical castration). Identifying a resource for the person to ask questions will help in allowing the patient to make the best decision for him. See chapter 5 for further information on the factors to consider during the decision-making process.

Each person going through hormone therapy will have different issues that are important to him. It is beneficial for the nurse to discuss these issues with the patient so that there is a mutual understanding of the primary goal and focus of the patient. This focus may change during the treatment, as the patient's situation changes. Helping the patient to identify what is important to him may help clarify issues for the patient.

Studies of patients on hormone therapy have focused on sexual functioning (Fitch et al., 2000), but recent clinical trials have begun to study QOL issues. One study looked at whether response to treatment for advanced prostate cancer impacted QOL and if nonresponders to treatment experienced a negative impact on QOL. Using questionnaires at several points during their treatment, 33 men participated in this study which showed that men who are responding to therapy will demonstrate improved QOL scores over those who do not respond, despite the toxicities of the treatment (Esper, Hamptom, Smith, & Pienta, 1999).

Patients have described living with the side effects of hormone therapy in a variety of ways. That description can range from "bothersome" to "severe" symptoms. In the latter case, the patient may consider stopping the treatment. Patients need to be told what is normal and what is outside the normal range so that they can alert health care professionals to potential problem areas. Fitch and colleagues (2000) found that many patients believe that they do not get the assistance that they need. Nurses working with these patients need to be alert to changes in a patient's condition so that interventions can be instituted to help the patient deal with the effects of the disease or the treatment.

The main side effect that men treated with hormone therapy complain about is hot flashes. Hot flashes are described as sudden sensations of heat felt in the face, neck, and chest that spread over the entire body. They are usually accompanied by profuse sweating and are followed by a chill. Hot flashes seem to be most bothersome when they occur at night and disturb sleep. While these often do not begin for several months following the start of hormone therapy, the degree of difficulty experienced by the men from the hot flashes can vary from minimal to intense. The severity of the hot flashes often decreases with time, and there is no intervention that is ideal for all patients. There are medications available that can help control the hot flashes. The use of Megace®, Catapres®, Depo-Provera®, or vitamin E has helped some men. However, many men resist the idea of taking additional medication to alleviate the side effects from the hormones. The main side effects of Megace (20 mg qd to qid) can be chills, appetite stimulation, and weight gain. Catapres (0.1 mg/day), an antihypertensive medication, can cause hypotension and skin reactions. Depo-Provera has no identified side effects when used every six months or less. Vitamin E, taken in 800 mg dosages, likewise has no identified side effects at this dosage, although patients should be told to stop this medication seven days prior to any surgical procedure since there is potential for bleeding while taking this medication. While none of these options guarantees to alleviate the hot flashes, men who are suffering from severe hot flashes do have these options available to them. These treatments may help to improve QOL by decreasing the discomfort caused by the hot flashes.

Decreased libido and impotence are other side effects of hormone therapy. These are the result of decreased testosterone and can have a significant impact on QOL, as well as on the person's perception of himself as a man. One patient described this as "being in a candy store and not being hungry." Many men believe that sexual activity is over when hormone therapy starts. Injection therapy, vacuum devices, and Viagra® (sildenafil) may work to help the patient have an erection, but the decreased libido is the prime issue. A discussion with the patient may help him to understand that there are other methods that can be used to remain close to and loving with his partner other than intercourse. Chapter 10 provides a further discussion on aspects of sexuality and intimacy pertinent to prostate cancer patients.

Fatigue is a common side effect that a patient may experience while on hormone therapy. It is usually not an early effect of the medication, but it can occur at some point. There are many reasons that a man on hormone therapy might experience fatigue, inadequate sleep or rest, pain, anemia, depression, or anxiety. The cause while on hormone therapy is most likely the suppression of testosterone. If the person is physically able, a program of regular exercise may help to increase his stamina and endurance to help fight the fatigue and maintain muscle mass (Stempkowski, 2000). It will also help with the weight gain (particularly around the hips and abdomen). The patient may think that the fatigue is caused by disease progression, so it is important to discuss the probable cause several times during the treatment to reinforce the cause. For a further discussion on fatigue, see chapter 7.

Osteoporosis is another late effect of hormone therapy. Androgens play an important role in bone metabolism. The relationship between the loss of estrogen and the development of osteoporosis has been well studied in women, and it has been identified as a potential problem in men on hormone therapy. There is not a significant difference in bone loss between men who have had a bilateral orchiectomy or men on LHRH agonists. Fosamax® may help to maintain bone density in the short term, but regular weight-bearing exercise may help to decrease bone density loss.

Gynecomastia and breast tenderness are side effects of the antiandrogens. Using over the counter pain medication when appropriate can help with the discomfort caused by the medication. Stopping the antiandrogen medication is the only other thing that can relieve this discomfort.

Prostate cancer support groups may be useful in helping men and their significant others cope with the effects of prostate cancer and the treatments. Patients can receive psychological support, encouragement, and reinforcement for what they are doing, along with information, at these meetings. A common perception is that a man does not share feelings and fears since our society dictates that men are "strong." Attending support groups can allow men to discover that others are experiencing similar feelings and concerns. It also gives the person going through this process the opportunity to help others.

There are many support groups available for men, including the *Man to Man* groups supported by the American Cancer Society and *Us Too International!,* groups founded by men with prostate cancer. Current research indicates that most men diagnosed with prostate cancer do not attend a support group for a variety of reasons (Krizek et al., 1999; Weber, Roberts, & McDougall, 2000).

When chemotherapy is being considered, patient education is essential. The patient needs to understand the goal of the treatment, the risks and the benefits, as well as other treatment options that might be available to him. Once the decision for chemotherapy is made, information on the specific chemotherapy agents should be given to the patient. Written information of the dosage schedule and possible side effects will help the patient to better understand what will occur. It will also help him to differentiate between side effects of the treatment and effects that are related to the disease. Nursing care and management of side effects of the patient receiving chemotherapy will depend upon the agents that the patient is receiving.

There are multiple side effects that can occur when a patient is receiving chemotherapy. Some examples include: edema, stomatitis, diarrhea, fever, chills, and hematuria. If the patient is educated about the likelihood of these effects, many can be managed by the patient, in conjunction with the nurse. Of vital importance is a resource person the patient can call when he needs help to determine when he needs medical evaluation or intervention for changes in his condition or treatment side effects. A nurse is pivotal in helping to identify situations that need intervention.

CONCLUSION

It is not easy to care for a patient with an incurable disease. There are many opportunities along the metastatic prostate cancer path that allow a nurse to help manage the disease, counsel, and support the patient and his family. These occasions not only help the patient, but they provide some of the most meaningful experiences in a nursing career.

The future for prostate cancer treatment is an open door. New and innovative methods are being studied and tried that prolong the life of the patient with metastatic prostate cancer. The quality of the patient's life during the treatment is also being studied and evaluated. The hope and dream is to both kill prostate cancer cells and do this in a way that allows the patient to maintain the quality in his life.

9

Watchful Waiting—Managing Prostate Cancer as a Chronic Disease

Meredith Wallace

The low mortality rate associated with prostate cancer and the high risks and costs associated with prostate cancer treatment have led some clinicians to choose not to aggressively treat, but rather to periodically observe patients. This treatment, known as "watchful waiting," "surveillance," or "expectant management" is defined as the use of no local or systemic therapy once prostate cancer has been diagnosed (Palmer & Chodak, 1996).

Watchful waiting takes factors such as age, other medical conditions, and tumor qualities into consideration in the decision of whether to treat, and how to treat prostate cancer. It is most appropriate for men whose life expectancy is less than 10 to 15 years and/or who have low-grade tumors. Naitoh, Zeiner, and DeKernion (1998) report that watchful waiting is an appropriate treatment and management option for prostate cancer in older patients or patients with other serious illnesses. The literature reveals that watchful waiting is primarily a treatment of older men.

Despite the low mortality associated with prostate cancer, aggressive forms of therapy for the disease have continued to supercede watchful waiting as a treatment option. In fact, only 13% of primary care physicians and 3% of urologists consider watchful waiting to be as appropriate as aggressive therapy (Fowler et al., 1998). In addition to physician preference, one study found that 22.4% of men surveyed would prefer aggressive treatment rather than watchful waiting even if their cancer was slow growing (Collins, Roberts, Oesterling, Wasson, & Barry, 1998).

Much attention has been paid to watchful waiting in the media. Men with prostate cancer and their families, as well as consumer's with concerns for where their healthcare dollars are being spent, are often subject to the media reports concerning this seemingly cost-effective strategy. Simple logic dictates that watchful waiting is less expensive than surgery, radiation or medications for the disease. However, despite, the large amount of media attention to this seemingly practical form of therapy, little research has been conducted to guide the experience of men who are receiving this approach. Gray, Fitch, Phillips, Labrecque, and Klotz (1999) report that "watchful waiting protocols require further study from a psychological perspective."

Men who are undergoing watchful waiting for prostate cancer are in need of clinical care by experienced and knowledgeable nurses. Care and teaching regarding the physical symptoms that are likely to accompany prostate cancer, as well as the psychological, emotional and family impacts of the disease, must be assessed and managed by the nurse. In addition, the role of uncertainty associated with living with prostate cancer for men, and the impact of uncertainty on aspects of quality of life must be explored by nurses.

This chapter will review the current literature on watchful waiting in men with prostate cancer, including descriptive studies of men receiving this treatment, the decision-making process, and mortality associated with this treatment. The clinical nursing care required of men who are watchful waiting, including necessary follow-up assessment of the disease and symptoms and uncertainty management will be discussed. The chapter will conclude with a discussion of the ethical and financial issues surrounding this treatment and future directions.

REVIEW OF LITERATURE

A Medline review from 1966 to present using the key words "watchful waiting" and "prostate cancer," resulted in only 85 articles. None of these articles was from a nursing perspective. Consequently, the current literature on this treatment option for prostate cancer is from a medical framework. This review of literature will be organized primarily around the two main areas identified in the search:

1. descriptive studies of characteristics of men undergoing watchful waiting and their providers;
2. treatment mortality.

CLINICAL AND PERSONAL CHARACTERISTICS OF WATCHFUL WAITERS

Men who are undergoing watchful waiting are likely to be older than most men diagnosed with prostate cancer, have other medical conditions and low-grade tumors. Watchful waiting is most appropriate for men whose life expectancy is less than 10 to 15 years. Naitoh, Zeiner, and DeKernion (1998) found it to be an appropriate treatment and management option for prostate cancer in older patients or patients with other serious illnesses that would threaten their lives more quickly than the prostate cancer.

Koppie and colleagues (2000) conducted a study to determine the demographic and clinical profile of men who elect watchful waiting as a management option by analyzing a database of 329 men undergoing watchful waiting from the Cancer of the Prostate Strategic Urological Research Endeavor (CaPSURE). Chi-square analysis revealed that patients managed with watchful waiting were more likely to be 75 years old or older and have a low serum PSA, organ-confined disease, and a total Gleason score of 7 or less.

The cohort of men who receive the watchful waiting management range significantly in their personal characteristics. Some men are very healthy despite their diagnosis of prostate cancer and have chosen to "watch" the disease. These men often reserve the right to choose more aggressive treatment if the tumor changes and causes pain, decreases in function, or risk of death. Other men who undergo the watchful waiting approach may have been diagnosed at a late stage and are therefore not candidates for aggressive therapy.

The decision to treat or not treat prostate cancer and watchfully await the disease is not an easy one. It is complicated by the fact that "no well-accepted, adequately powered randomized trial of competing modalities for this disease has ever been completed" (Walther, 1999). Consequently, many factors must be considered when determining whether to select an aggressive or nonaggressive route to managing the disease. For further information on factors involved in the decision-making process refer to chapter 4.

As mentioned earlier, age and size of the tumor are two important factors in choosing a treatment approach. One study of 1,809 men diagnosed with prostate cancer during a screening, indicated that 79.2% chose radical prostatectomy, 12.4% chose radiation therapy, and 8.4% chose watchful waiting as their primary treatment. Further analyses revealed that education, income, age, indication for prostate biopsy, comorbidity score, serum PSA level, clinical stage, and pretreatment urinary and sexual function were associated significantly with treatment choice, but race, marital status, and Gleason grade were not. Furthermore, for every five year decrease in age, the odds for choosing radiation over watchful waiting increased (Yan, Carvalhal, Catalona, & Young, 2000).

Mazur and Hickam (1996) interviewed 140 men with a mean age of 66.3 years to determine whether patients with early localized prostate cancer would prefer surgery over watchful waiting, and why. Of the 140 patients, 53% preferred surgical treatment, 42% preferred watchful waiting, and only 4% preferred that their physician make the decision. Of those electing surgery, the majority believed that the curative nature of the procedure had the strongest influence on their decision.

Physician treatment preference plays a large role in the choice of therapy a man receives. Fowler and colleagues (2000) conducted a mailed survey of 504 urologists and radiation oncologists to determine physician treatment patterns. For men with moderately differentiated, clinically localized cancers, and a more than 10-year life expectancy, 93% of urologists chose radical prostatectomy. Both urologists and radiation oncologists were significantly more likely to recommend the treatment in their specialty than the other treatment (i.e., radical prostatectomy and radiation therapy, respectively). Neither group preferred watchful waiting except men with life expectancies of less than 10 years, and cancers with very favorable prognoses.

Overall, the decision on how to treat prostate cancer is complex and includes the consideration of many factors. The Prostate Outcomes Research Team (PORT) designed a model to explore the effect of treatment for localized prostate cancer on the morbidity and mortality of the disease to aide in the treatment decision (Fleming, Wasson, Albertsen, Barry, & Wennberg, 1993). Three options were explored; radical prostatectomy, external-beam radiation therapy, and watchful waiting, with delayed hormonal therapy if metastatic disease develops. The model was tested on men aged 60 to 75 with well, moderately, and poorly differentiated prostate cancers. The results showed that radical prostatectomy and radiation therapy are beneficial in reducing morbidity and mortality among patients with localized prostate cancer, particularly younger patients with higher-grade tumors. However, the model showed that in most cases the potential benefit of treatment in reducing morbidity and mortality of disease was small enough that the choice of therapy is relatively inconsequential. The team concluded that watchful waiting is a reasonable alternative to aggressive treatment for many men with prostate cancer.

Clinical and personal indicators commonly found in the literature and included in the decision-making process are summarized in Table 9.1. These factors, as well as the patient characteristics, remain the hallmark of

TABLE 9.1 Personal and Clinical Characteristics of Men Who are Receiving the Watchful Waiting Treatment

- life expectancy less than 10 to 15 years
- 70 years old or older
- significant co-morbidity
- low grade tumors
- lower serum PSA
- organ confined disease
- total Gleason score of 7 or less
- urinary and sexual dysfunction

the decision-making process, However, patient and physician preference for treatment plays a large role in the decision. These factors of the decision-making process require further study.

MORTALITY ASSOCIATED WITH WATCHFUL WAITING

A major factor influencing the decision to aggressively treat prostate cancer or choose watchful waiting lies in the prognosis of the disease. At this time, personal characteristics and clinical factors such as age and tumor size appear to hold the greatest weight in making that decision. However, knowing how long the person will live after a diagnosis of prostate cancer, and the influence it will have on quality of life, are important considerations in making the treatment decision.

Several studies have been conducted on the mortality of men receiving the watchful waiting treatment. In a Swedish study of 233 older men with early stage prostate cancer, given no initial treatment, only 19 men died of prostate cancer, after 10 years, whereas 105 died of other causes. (Johansson et al., 1992). However, Palmer and Chodak (1996) report that studies are methodologically inconsistent. Specifically, numerical values assigned to side effects of treatments were chosen arbitrarily. Palmer and Chodak (1996) summarized that "the studies reported a rather low risk of dying from prostate cancer in 10 years for all but poorly differentiated cancers" (p. 552).

Albertson and colleagues (1995) conducted a study of 65- to 75-year old men who were receiving the watchful waiting treatment for prostate cancer. He found the 10-year cancer specific survival rate was 91%, 76%, and 52%, respectively, for men with well differentiated, moderately differentiated and poorly differentiated cancers, and the 15-year survival to be 72% for well differentiated cancers and 48% for moderately and poorly differentiated cancers.

Neulander, Duncan, Tiguert, Posey, and Soloway (2000) assessed the effect of clinical stage, Gleason score, change in PSA score, and age, on the progression of disease of 54 men with a mean age 76.4 years, who were undergoing watchful waiting. Of the 54 patients, 28 (52%) experienced a progression of the disease. The mean time to progression was 35 months. Using multivariate analysis, Gleason score and PSA level were statistically significant predictors of disease progression. The small sample size of this study limits the generalizability of the findings. However, the study provides further information to support the consideration of Gleason score and PSA as two clinical indicators that may be helpful in determining individual patient prognosis and aide in the decision-making process.

Several researchers are exploring prospective ways in which to predict mortality using clinical indicators. Borre, Offersen, Nerstrom, and Overgaard (1998) examined angiogenesis, the formation of new blood vessels, as a method to provide important prognostic information to assist in the decision-making process regarding prostate cancer. Angiogenesis was assessed in a sample of 221 men who were undergoing watchful waiting, by looking at the microvessel density at diagnosis and again at death. The median length of follow-up was 15 years. Microvessal density was significantly related to clinical stage of prostate cancer and histological grade and significantly predicted survival in the sample. In a secondary analysis of the sample, Borre, Nerstrom, and Overgaard (2000) found that all of the tumors exhibited cytoplasmic staining for vascular endothelial growth factor of neuroendocrine-differentiated tumor cells. This study offers promise for further investigation of factors that may determine the prognosis of the patient with prostate cancer and aid in the decision on how to treat the disease.

Grover and associates (2000) investigated the mortality of men treated for prostate cancer. The researchers analyzed 59,000 cases in a prostate cancer database for the incidence of age-specific prostate cancer, distribution of diagnosed tumors, according to patient age, clinical stage and tumor grade, initial treatment, treatment complications, and progression to metastatic disease and death. The data were used to validate a model designed to calculate age, stage, tumor grade, and treatment-specific clinical outcomes of men with prostate cancer. The results revealed support for the ability of the model to forecast clinical outcomes for individual men who have prostate cancer or are at risk for the disease. Further research is needed on the morbidity and mortality of men who receive the watchful waiting management option in order for its role in the treatment decision-making process to become more readily understood.

CLINICAL NURSING MANAGEMENT OF WATCHFUL WAITING PATIENTS

Clinical nursing management of patients who undergo the watchful waiting option focuses on several dimensions of quality of life (QOL). Physical function including, consideration of medical follow-up, medications and interventions to control symptoms of the disease, including altered sexual and urinary functioning and pain are of large concern to the nurse. Well-being focuses on the uncertainty surrounding the progression of the disease within this treatment approach to prostate cancer, and has an effect on the overall QOL of the patient and family. The following section of this chapter will address these dimensions and the nursing care necessary to maintain optimal function and well-being.

Assessment

An essential component of nursing care for the man who is receiving the watchful waiting treatment is continual evaluation of the growth of the prostate cancer tumor. While most men who undergo the watchful waiting approach likely have clinically localized disease, men with all tumor grades may consider this option. Therefore, vigilant observation for the progression of both local and systemic disease is warranted. Two methods are found to be most prevalent in monitoring the growth of the tumor; PSA blood levels and digital rectal examination (DRE) of the gland (Carter & Partin, 1998). When necessary, transrectal ultrasound (TRUS) of the prostate gland may also be used to assess tumor growth.

PSA evaluation should be conducted every six months in patients receiving the watchful waiting treatment. Nam, Klotz, Jewett, Danjoux, and Trachtenberg (1998) studied the rate of change in PSA in men with prostate cancer initially managed by watchful waiting. PSA levels were determined in 74 subjects with a mean age of 69 years. The results showed that the PSA of the sample rose rapidly 31% of the time. This finding suggests that evaluating PSA levels less than every six months may falsely indicate disease progression.

Evaluation of tumor growth may be made most effectively by DRE. DRE is the most cost-effective and clinically supported method for determining a change in the tumor. DRE involves manual palpation of the prostate gland through the rectal wall. Documentation of the symmetry of the gland, induration and presence and location of nodules may be most effectively completed on a drawing of the prostate gland. The results of successive DRE should be compared to determine a clinical picture of the disease progression. (Refer to chapter 3 for further information on DRE.)

Transrectal ultrasound of the prostate gland (TRUS), often accompanied by needle biopsy, may be used as a diagnostic tool. Naryayan (1995) reports that TRUS is a useful tool to evaluate the prostate gland and to determine the size and location of the tumor. Lee and colleagues (1988) report that the sensitivity rate of TRUS is twice that of DRE in detecting prostate tumors. However, Pobursky (1995) reports that TRUS is expensive and has limited value in staging prostate cancer that has already been diagnosed. He further reports, however, that if seminal vesicle invasion is suspected, TRUS is an effective method of detection.

Evaluation of the symptoms of prostate cancer should be part of the patient evaluation conducted every six months. Symptoms of the disease generally relate to sexual and urinary function. One way to effectively evaluate symptoms is by using a standardized quantitative prostate cancer inventory (see Figure 9.1). By quantitatively measuring the symptoms of the disease, numerical scores can be compared to effectively determine symptom progression.

MANAGEMENT

A great deal of teaching by the nurse is necessary for patients who are receiving watchful waiting, particularly surrounding the decision-making process. Individuals must be provided with both the positive and negative aspects of this treatment approach. It is necessary to talk with the patient and family making the decision, about treatment side effects, and overall treatment costs associated with this form of therapy. The risk of tumor growth and metatasis, potential pain, alteration in function and quality of life, and shortened lifespan, all must be explored. During the decision-making process it is important to assure the patient that watchful waiting does not mean that he will be ignored as a patient. The risks and benefits, as revealed in the literature surrounding watchful waiting, are summarized in Table 9.2. If treatment becomes necessary to prevent the spread of the disease in the future, the patient must be assured that this will be given full consideration.

Uncertainty

Uncertainty is defined as the "inability to determine the meaning of illness-related events which occurs in situations where the decision maker is unable to assign definite values to objects and events and/or is unable to accurately predict outcomes because sufficient cues are lacking" (Mishel, 1988, p. 225). It has been determined to be a major stressor for patients coping with life-threatening illnesses (Mishel, 1988). Specifically, evidence has shown that uncertainty plays an important role in the lives of men who are aggressively treated for prostate cancer with radical

	Never	Sometimes	Often	Always
Please choose the best answer.				
In the past month, how often have you noticed:				
1. Weak urinary stream	___	___	___	___
2. Difficulty urinating	___	___	___	___
3. Blood in semen	___	___	___	___
4. Blood stains on underwear	___	___	___	___
5. Frequent urination	___	___	___	___
6. Urinary urgency	___	___	___	___
7. Straining or pushing while urinating	___	___	___	___
8. Blood in urine	___	___	___	___
9. Pain or burning when urinating	___	___	___	___
10. Discharge on underwear	___	___	___	___
11. Sensation of incomplete bladder emptying	___	___	___	___
12. Need to urinate at night	___	___	___	___

Note. The validity and reliability of this instrument was supported in a study of 19 men who were receiving the watchful waiting treatment (Wallace, 2001). Each symptom is assessed with a four-point Likert scale ranging from almost never "0" to almost always "3." The maximum score, indicating high symptomatology, is 3.

FIGURE 9.1 Wallace Prostate Cancer Symptom Inventory.

prostatectomy or radiation (Germino et al., 1998). Men who are undergoing the watchful waiting for prostate cancer may have uncertainty about the disease that extends throughout their lives. However, the role of uncertainty in men undergoing the watchful waiting management approach to prostate cancer has only recently been examined.

TABLE 9.2 Risks and Benefits of the Watchful Waiting Treatment for Prostate Cancer

Risks	Benefits
• noncurative • changeover to life-threatening disease is possible • pain, decreased sexual and urinary function if disease progresses	• lower cost • no side effects of treatment • aggressive treatment may be considered at a later date

A descriptive study, conducted by Wallace (2001), indicated that uncertainty explained approximately 36% of the variance in QOL among 19 older men receiving the watchful waiting treatment for prostate cancer. Specifically, the results of the study revealed that uncertainty predicted well-being as a dimension of QOL.

Mishel and colleagues (personal communication, Mishel, October, 1999) are currently conducting a multi-site study funded by the National Institute of Nursing Research, based on the predicted impact of uncertainty on outcomes of prostate cancer. Based on previous theoretical work with the concept, an intervention program, entitled "Uncertainty Management Intervention," has been developed. In this program nurses provide follow-up care to prostate cancer patients with unanswered concerns regarding their radiation and surgery treatment (watchful waiting patients were not included in this study). The nurses make one telephone call per week for six weeks at a scheduled date and time. Although statistical analyses have not yet been published, early results of four clinical trials have shown a reduction in the number of patient problems, including incontinent episodes and other disease-related symptoms. In addition, the promotion of self-advocacy for care, family relationships, and QOL have improved as a result of this nursing intervention.

While this is an excellent beginning, the relationship between uncertainty resulting from living with prostate cancer requires additional research. The fear of cancer resulting in death and disability among older adults, in conjunction with demonstrated low QOL in men who are receiving the watchful waiting treatment for prostate cancer, lends further support to the need to manage uncertainty in this population.

Family Support

The patient's wife or significant other, other family members, and friends may have many feelings regarding the patient's diagnosis of prostate cancer and his treatment choice. Further counseling by the nurse may be provided to include the family and significant others when possible. At this time, the family members may bring forth their questions and concerns regarding the diagnosis and treatment choice. It is very important for the patient's family and significant others to understand and to accept the decision of the patient about his treatment. However, if no agreement can be reached that is amenable to both the patient and family, the patient's needs and wishes must be the nurse's primary consideration.

Symptom Management

As the tumor progresses in size, pressure is often placed on the surrounding urinary and reproductive structures. This pressure may result in alteration of function and pain. Problems with urination are common among men who are receiving the watchful waiting treatment. Urinary retention may be seen as a problem in men who are watchful waiting and should be evaluated. See chapter 7 for an in-depth description of diagnosing and managing urinary retention.

Although the need to express sexuality continues throughout the lifespan, men with prostate cancer may experience an alteration in sexual functioning. Problems with sexual functioning are common among men who are watchful waiting. In a study of 19 subjects, sexual function, as measured by the University of California Prostate Cancer Inventory (UCLA-PCI) received a mean score of 41%, indicating poor sexual function (Wallace, 2001). Problems reported by the sample included difficulty in developing and maintaining an erection.

A sexual assessment provides nurses with information to assist at an early point to prevent or correct sexual problems. The PLISSIT model has been used to assess and to manage the sexuality of adults (Annon, 1976). The model includes obtaining permission from the client to initiate sexual discussion (*P*), providing the limited information needed to function sexually (*LI*), giving specific suggestions for the individual to proceed with sexual relations (*SS*), and providing intensive therapy surrounding the issues of sexuality for that client (*IT*). It is common for nurses to feel uncomfortable with assessing the sexual desires and functions of clients. Regardless, a sexual assessment should be performed as a routine part of the nursing assessment. Knowledge, skill, and a sense of comfort is necessary for the nurse to assess sexuality. Skill and a sense of comfort in assessing sexuality comes with practice (Billhorn, 1994).

Currently, erectogenic agents such as Viagra®, are available to assist the man with prostate cancer to develop and maintain an erection. Although no studies could be found to support the use of this medication in the watchful waiting population, the smooth muscle relaxation and improved blood flow achieved by the medication may be effective at improving their sexual function. Vacuum constriction devices (VCD) may also be an option to explore for men experiencing erectile problems as a result of tumor pressure on the reproductive structures.

When sexual intercourse is not the preferred method of intimacy or is not possible, the couple may be taught alternative methods of intimacy in the form of touch. Kaplan (1990) recommends that a oriented sex therapy program focused on intimacy will result in improved sexuality. Touch is a means of expressing intimacy and closeness that may fulfill the sexual needs and desires of older clients. Touch can best be fulfilled by acquiring a comfortable environment in which the adult couple can expose parts of their bodies to each other as they feel comfortable. A shower or bath may be enjoyable. The couple should be taught to slowly or lightly move their fingertips over each other's skin while enjoying the closeness of the other person. Massage therapy books and videos may provide the gentleman and his partner with a way in which to provide touch that results in the fulfillment of sexual desires. Soft music may add to creating a conducive environment for the couple.

With tumor growth, one of the first signs may be pain. Pain may cause the client to seek medical care and a change of treatment. However, if aggressive treatment to reduce the tumor is not received, chronic pain may become a problem for men who are watchful waiting. Chronic pain results in depression, decreased socialization, sleep disturbances, impaired ambulation, and increased healthcare utilization and costs (American Geriatric Society [AGS], 1998). Pain assessment and management are paramount in providing nursing care to men with prostate cancer and preventing the consequences of pain. However, the detection and management of pain is complex and must include routine pain assessment, diagnosis, the careful use of analgesic drugs, and the utilization of non-pharmacological approaches such as physical therapy interventions and non-traditional approaches. For a comprehensive discussion of pain assessment, see chapter 11.

Treatment of pain usually involves the administration of medication. However, since watchful waiting is primarily an option of older adults, it is important to note that managing pain in the elderly through the use of pharmacological interventions is complicated by adverse reactions and analgesic sensitivity. Popp and Portenoy (1996) report that safe, effective use of analgesic drugs in the elderly requires in-depth knowledge of age-related changes in pharmacokinetics and pharmacodynamics. The old adage "start low and go slow" (AGS, 1998) is an appropriate rule for administration of pain medications in older adults.

Non-opioid pain management, primarily acetaminophen and non-steroidal anti-inflammatory drugs (NSAIDs) in the older population are the first line of treatment for pain. These medications should be used discriminately in this population because of the risk of side effects. Skander and Ryan (1988) report a descriptive study of two groups of patients, aged 65 to 74 and 75 and over, visualized during endoscopy to assess for the presence of ulcers. Results correlated with a history of NSAID use for the six weeks preceding the procedure, revealed NSAIDs contribute to ulceration and mask pain that leads to ulcer diagnosis. The addition of misoprostol, histamin-2-receptor antagonists, proton pump inhibitors, and antacids have been supported as adjuncts to NSAIDs in the elderly. However, these medications are not entirely effective in alleviating the risk of side effects with NSAID use (AGS, 1998). Protective medications are not without effects and the harm must be weighed against the potential benefit. NSAIDs should be used with caution in older adults and may be replaced by acetaminophen when appropriate because of the high risk of renal and gastrointestinal side effects in the older population.

As pain progresses, the administration of opioids for effective management may be necessary. Opioids are effective in controlling pain. Moreover, Ferrell, Wisdom, Wenzl, and Brown (1989), in a study of 83 subjects randomly assigned to receive either MS-Contin or a short-acting analgesic, concluded that through appropriate pain management with pain therapies such as controlled-release analgesics, nurses can greatly enhance QOL for cancer patients. However, studies suggest the need to decrease morphine dosages in older patients (AGS, 1998). Therefore, it is recommended that older patients be managed on an individual basis, titrating dose and frequency according to the requirements of the patient. Age should be used as a factor in choosing initial dosing frequency.

The use of nonpharmacological methods of pain management have increased over the past several years. Biofeedback, guided imagery, exercise, and relaxation have all been supported as effective alternative methods of acute and chronic pain management. Further research is needed on the application of these techniques to the man experiencing prostate cancer pain.

ECONOMIC, ETHICAL CONCERNS, FUNDING ISSUES, AND FUTURE DIRECTIONS

Prostate cancer, one of the leading causes of cancer in older men, is a prevalent problem that impacts the lives of individuals, health care providers, politicians, researchers, private industries, environmentalists, and many other groups of citizens. To attempt to develop commentary on how each of these groups of individuals are effected by the disease and the choice of treatment, is beyond the scope of this chapter. However, no discussion of the watchful waiting treatment would be complete without exploring the prevalent beliefs among healthcare professionals and society that prevent the full acceptance of this form of disease management.

It is generally believed that people cannot live a quality life with a cancerous growth within their body. This leads to the need to eradicate the disease with aggressive treatment and at high costs to both patients and tax payers. Since it is clear that the watch and wait approach to prostate cancer is much less expensive than more aggressive surgical or radiation treatments, it is time to derive an expanded understanding of watchful waiting on quality of life. Such an analysis may save medical dollars by allowing men to live high-quality lives with prostate cancer. Providing quality nursing care in the form of teaching and state of the art assessment and management may substantially contribute to the QOL of older adults and eventually influence the ability of policy makers to save money by discouraging aggressive treatments unless more conservative approaches are first discussed.

In summary, watchful waiting is an appropriate treatment choice for older men with certain clinical indicators (see Table 9.1). Approximately 11% of all men with prostate cancer receive watchful waiting. The literature describing this management option is primarily focused on profiling the patient with this form of treatment, the decision-making process and the mortality of the disease. Little information is available to guide the nursing care of men who watch and wait. This chapter provides the reader with information on the assessment, management and teaching regarding the physical symptoms that are likely to accompany prostate cancer, as well as the psychological, emotional and family impacts of the disease. Men who are receiving the watchful waiting approach to prostate cancer are in need of clinical care by experienced and knowledgeable nurses. The chronic character of prostate cancer must be acknowledged, and further research on the most effective methods of care for this population are needed. Only when these two areas are fully examined, will further information become available to view watchful waiting as a more viable option for management of prostate cancer.

10
Prevalent Issues in Patient Education

Vanna M. Dest and Meredith Wallace

Throughout the assessment, diagnosis, and treatment of prostate cancer, patients and families require continued education. The relationship of the symptoms to the disease, the procedures aimed at diagnosis, and the various treatment options require that much information be obtained on by the consumer. In the case of prostate cancer, it is often the role of nurses to provide this information to the patients and their loved ones in an understandable format.

There has been much written about patient education in the nursing literature. Health education is a major focus of the United States Department of Health & Human Services Healthy People 2010: National Health-Promotion and Disease-Prevention Objectives *(http://www.health.gov/healthypeople)*. While the need to educate may be clearly understood, the process is often difficult. Teaching at the time of diagnosis or a procedure is not often successful and the information is readily lost. Teaching through discussion and written information is most effective. This combination of methods allows the patient and family to focus on their needs at a later time, when thinking may be clearer. Asking follow-up questions to determine understanding of the information, is a valuable method in which to evaluate the effectiveness of teaching and to assist in planning future educational sessions.

While each chapter in this book has addressed the information needs particular to issues in prostate cancer and treatment choice, this chapter will address several important areas in which men require in-depth understanding in order for effective management to result. Specifically, urinary and sexual function are discussed. The chapter concludes with a discussion on the family's role in disease management.

PATIENT AND FAMILY EDUCATION

Patient and family education are key components in the care of the prostate cancer patient. Education is the mechanism by which information is provided to patients and their families. The positive outcomes of patient education include increased compliance with treatment, self-care activities to manage side effects, strategies for fewer side effects, and improved coping skills with disease and its treatment (Sporkin, 1992). It is important to keep in mind that patient educational goals related to prostate cancer treatment may vary from the goals of health care professionals. In order to determine the needs of the patient, nurses must assess the learning needs of the patient, readiness to learn, and factors that may affect the ability to learn. Factors that may affect the ability to learn include the patient's own personal expectations of prostate cancer treatment, which may include misconceptions and fears about treatment, cultural beliefs, language barriers, level of literacy, and concomitant physical or psychosocial symptoms such as pain, fatigue, anxiety, or depression. Fears and misconceptions about treatment should be addressed prior to initiating an educational plan. Some common misconceptions of radiation therapy include fear of being radioactive, "horror stories" associated with older, less advanced technology, such as cobalt therapy, and belief that radiation therapy is a last resort treatment. Fears of radical prostatectomy include loss of manhood and subsequent virility. In addition, men who are receiving the watchful waiting treatment often fear random disease progression. As nurses, it is important to set learning goals and provide information that is appropriate to individual patients and families. Goals which are indicated in the cancer population include the provision of knowledge and facts, the development of self-care activities, and the support of desired attitudes and behaviors (Lindeman, 1988). Villejo and Meyers (1991) found that providing patients and their families with information about the disease and treatment helped to increase their coping and gaining a sense of control over a virtually uncontrollable situation.

It is also important to consider that the educational needs of patients and families may change throughout the cancer journey and its different phases. For example, five different phases are identified and include the diagnostic phase, treatment phase, rehabilitation or continuing care phase, cancer survivorship or remission phase, and recurrence or advanced disease phase (Adams, 1991). During the diagnostic phase, patients require information regarding diagnostic tests, potential problems, and the differential diagnoses. Diagnostic tests for prostate cancer may include PSA, transrectal ultrasound guided biopsy of the prostate gland (TRUS), computed axial tomography (CAT) scan of the abdomen and pelvis with or without contrast, radionuclide bone scan, magnetic resonance imaging (MRI) of the pelvis, and plain x-rays.

During the treatment phase, patients and their families are dealing with information about the type of cancer, extent of disease, patterns of spread or metastasis, appropriate treatment options, and their associated side effects and prognosis. In order for patients to make an informed decision they must gather information about the proposed treatment modality, side effects of treatment, sequence of treatment events (i.e., simulation, start of treatment, and follow-up), response and survival rates, prognosis, and rehabilitation and self-care activities (Crosson, 1984).

During the patient's initial consultation, the health care team provides detailed information regarding disease and prognosis with emphasis on appropriate treatment options, associated side effects, and complications and self-care activities. Patients should be told about the day to day routine of receiving treatment as well as the follow-up testing needed and anticipated side effects and interventions to manage them. This information may be overwhelming, therefore it is recommended that it be reinforced throughout the course of treatment.

Ideally, the rehabilitation phase should begin at the time of diagnosis. It should be centered on the goal of optimal functioning, which is dictated by the cancer itself and limitations that it may impose. With the changing direction of health care in the past decade from inpatient to outpatient services, there is even a greater need for education of self-care activities. In respect to self-care activities, Dodd (1984) evaluated the benefits of teaching patients about expected side effects and related self-care activities. Her research showed that patients who learned side effect management techniques for RT and chemotherapy performed more self-care activities and initiated them sooner than those not informed of self-care activities. For the patient with prostate cancer, rehabilitation issues may include learning to adapt and cope with fatigue, urinary symptoms such as frequency, nocturia, urgency, and dysuria, bowel problems and sexual dysfunction. Education during this phase should be geared toward enhancing quality of life and informing the patient and their families about community resources, such as home care, support groups, and complementary therapies (i.e., yoga, guided imagery, art therapy, hypnosis, and biofeedback).

The cancer survivorship phase begins at the time of diagnosis and continues throughout the cancer trajectory. Common feelings that cancer patients experience during this phase include fear of cancer recurrence, learning to live with the limitations and losses of cancer and its treatment, financial burden, survivor guilt, and social isolation from family members and friends (Zampini & Ostroff, 1993). In addition, issues of job and insurance discrimination can surface after a cancer diagnosis. Educating patients about support groups and organizations such as the American Cancer Society (ACS), the National Cancer Institute (NCI), Cancer Care Inc., and the National Coalition of Cancer Survivors

(NCCS) can be extremely beneficial in dealing with the issues of survivorship. In 1998, the Oncology Nursing Society (ONS), the Association of Oncology Social Workers (AOSW), and the National Coalition of Cancer Survivors (NCCS) developed a series of learning audiocassettes called the Cancer Survivor Toolbox. The toolbox focuses on learning skills related to communication, information seeking, decision making, problem solving, negotiating health care, and patient rights. Recent additions to the toolbox include financial matters and issues specific to the elderly population.

The last phase of the cancer journey is the recurrence or advanced disease phase. Many researchers believe that this is as difficult and very different from the initial diagnosis of cancer for both patients and families (Holland & Lewis, 2000; Mahon & Casperson, 1997). Although learning needs may be the same as those experienced during the diagnostic phase, they are often intensified because of treatment failure, poor prognosis and debilitation of disease. Feelings associated with recurrence can magnify issues of mortality, anger, grief, and uncertainty. Educational needs increase for family members and are commonly centered on symptom management, pain control and quality of life issues. Information about community resources such as home care, palliative care, and hospice may be appropriate. Patients with recurrent or metastatic prostate cancer face issues of treatment failure and the focus of treatment changes to controlling disease and comfort measures with the use of hormonal therapy, chemotherapy, RT, and pain management. Radiation therapy can also be utilized to alleviate or minimize bone pain with the use of external beam irradiation and/or radiopharmaceuticals such as Strontium-89 (Metastron®) or Samarium-153 (Quadramet®).

Regardless of the type of information provided to patients and family members, written information to supplement patient and family education is also very beneficial. Researchers have found that written information in combination with other forms of teaching increases patient knowledge (Frank-Stromborg & Cohen, 1991; Whitman-Obert, 1996). It is also important to inform patients and families about resources that can complement information regarding treatment options, side effects of treatment, and psychosocial issues. These include organizations such as the ACS, the NCI, and respected and reputable Internet web sites. The process of education is ongoing, beginning with the initial consultation, through the treatment, discharge, and follow-up period.

URINARY INCONTINENCE IN THE PATIENT WITH PROSTATE CANCER

The primary type of urinary dysfunction associated with prostate cancer is urinary incontinence (UI). UI, defined as the involuntary loss of urine, is recognized as both a major symptom of prostate cancer and side effect of disease treatment. The presence of UI often has far-reaching effects on men. These effects include: impaired skin integrity (Adamson, 1996), and decreased self-esteem. In addition, incontinent men fear accidents when away from home. Consequently they tend to avoid physical and social activities because of this problem, leading to social isolation.

Despite the high prevalence of the problem, men are hesitant to seek assistance with UI among healthcare providers. Lack of reporting may be due to embarrassment or acceptance of incontinence as a normal aging change or permanent side-effect of treatment. It is important for continued health and self-esteem for both patients and clinicians to accept incontinence as a manageable problem and seek treatment.

Assessing UI is the first step to appropriate management of the symptom or treatment side effect. The bladder diary is the recommended tool to collect information regarding UI. A sample bladder diary is provided in Figure 10.1. The diary may be provided to the patient to keep a log of the incontinent episodes as they occur throughout the day and night and associated environmental factors. In addition, sample screening questions are discussed in Figure 10.1. The diary and questions provide a framework for guiding assessment of presence and risk of incontinence. This information may be used by health care providers to determine the amplitude of the problem and guide appropriate symptom management.

While bladder diaries and suggested questions and screening frameworks help to identify the risk and presence of UI, these instruments do not shed light on the impact of incontinence on an individual's quality of life. The impact of UI on quality of life may vary based on whether it occurred as a symptom of the disease or treatment side-effect and the length of the UI. To assess the impact of UI, health care providers may choose an appropriate Health Related Quality of Life (HRQOL) instrument that measures specific UI symptomatology. Many HRQOLs are available, including the well-studied SF-36 (Ware & Sherbourne, 1992). In addition, Litwin and colleagues (1995) have adapted the SF-36 for prostate cancer into a new instrument, entitled the University of California at Los Angeles—Prostate Cancer Inventory (UCLA-PCI). This instrument includes a urinary-specific module. The results of HR-QOL instrument may shed further light on the impact of incontinence and guide management strategies.

Patient teaching regarding UI is a primary nursing responsibility. Patients and families must be assured that interventions are available to assist them with UI while living with prostate cancer or post-treatment. Assuring the patient and family that the nurse will thoroughly assess the problem and work with them until it is resolved is an essential first step in symptom management.

Patient Education

Do you ever lose control of your urine? Do you ever leak?

Can you tell me about the problems you are having with your bladder?

Can you tell me about the trouble you are having holding your urine (water)?

How often do you lose urine when you do not want to?

When do you lose urine when you do not want to?
  Do you leak when coughing, sneezing, laughing, or lifting objects? (Stress)
  Do you leak when hurrying to the bathroom?

How often do you wear a pad, diaper, undergarment-shield?

Do you use any other type of protection from leaking urine?

How long has this bladder problem been?

SAMPLE BLADDER RECORD—Should track a 24-hour time period for several days

Time Interval	Urinated in Toilet	Incontinent Episode (+ = small; +++ = large)	Reason for Incontinent Episode	Type and Amount of Liquid Intake	Bowel Movement	Pad/Diaper Use
7–8AM						
8–9AM						

Continue for a 24 hour time frame.

May also include a comment area.

Note. Adapted with permission from Castranova, A. M. (2001). Urinary incontinence. In *TRY THIS—Best Practice for Geriatric Nursing* (M. Wallace, Ed). Volume 2, Number 5. John A. Hartford Foundation Institute for Geriatric Nursing.

FIGURE 10.1 Suggested Questions to Guide Incontinence Assessment.

Baum, Appell, and Moss (1994) report that there are three different types of incontinence; stress incontinence, overflow incontinence and urge incontinence. Stress incontinence occurs during exercise, laughing, coughing, or sneezing. This type of incontinence occurs as the muscles supporting the bladder and surrounding structures become weak. For stress incontinence, Kegel exercises are often regarded as an effective treatment method. However the use of Kegel exercises in men with prostate cancer is controversial and further research is needed regarding the effectiveness of this intervention with prostate cancer patients. Overflow incontinence is caused by an enlarged prostate gland and will likely require surgical treatment.

The most common type of incontinence for men with prostate cancer is called urge incontinence. This type of incontinent symptom is manifested by the inability to delay voiding once the bladder is full. For men experiencing urge incontinence, regular toileting or habit training is encouraged. This is most effectively done when the man can select specific times during the day when he urinates. The bladder diary, displayed in Figure 10.1, is an effective tool in determining voiding times. After developing a schedule, the client should be instructed to use the toilet half an hour before this time each day. This technique may prevent incontinent episodes from occurring. Prompted voiding is another method to decrease incontinent episodes. The gentleman is reminded or asked by a family member, health care provider or significant other about voiding. A more structured bladder-training program allows individuals to develop a voiding schedule that is progressive, by increasing the time between voids and ensuring that adequate fluids are taken from 7 AM to 7 PM. Postponing voids by using relaxation, imagery, or distraction is essential to the success of this management strategy. This type of training is difficult and relies on a good working relationship between the individual, their family and the nurse. There are several medications available to reduce urge incontinence by relaxing the smooth muscle structures. These include Detrol® (tolerodine tartrate), Ditropan® (oxybutynin chloride), Tofranil® (imipramine hydrochloride), Pro-Banthine® (propantheline bromide), and dicyclomide hydrochloride.

UI is a common treatment side effect of prostate cancer. The presence of UI in men with prostate cancer often has devastating effects on health and self-esteem. It is an important nursing role to assure patients that UI is treatable. Nurses must work with patients using the interventions suggested to manage incontinence. Appropriate symptom management will help to prevent the sequelae of the symptom and allow the man with prostate cancer to live the highest possible quality of life.

SEXUAL DYSFUNCTION IN THE PATIENT WITH PROSTATE CANCER

Sexual dysfunction is a major problem in men with prostate cancer. The World Health Organization (1976) defines sexuality as the integration of somatic, emotional, intellectual, and social aspects of sexual being in ways that are positively enriching and that enhance personality, communication, and love. Sexuality is an integral part of an individual's personality.

Despite the continuing sexual interests and desires of men with prostate cancer, and the need for assistance in this area, few interventions are implemented by health care professionals to facilitate the expression of sexuality. Several reasons account for this lack of implementation. The most obvious continues to be society's distaste for and lack of insight into the sexual behavior of older men with prostate cancer. Kain, Reilly, and Schultz (1990) report that society's views on sexual behavior of older individuals are primarily negative and that such views inhibit the expression of sexuality among older adults. The thought of older, often disabled people engaging in sexual intercourse is not appealing to society. Nurses are also susceptible to society's myths and anxieties toward the sexual expressions of older men. A nurse's basic discomfort with sexuality issues may actually distort his or her perceptions of clients' needs (Drench & Losee, 1996). Opposing moral values may also add to the nursing staff's reluctance to intervene and to facilitate the sexual satisfaction of older adults.

Hillman and Stricker (1994) report that another reason why nurses do not intervene and facilitate the expression of sexuality is because they lack the knowledge and training to do so. Furthermore, they report that nursing programs generally do not provide adequate clinical training in the area of sexual desires and functioning. Without such training and experience, nurses are not confident enough to begin sensitive discussions about intimacy and sexuality.

Patient teaching regarding the common problems associated with prostate cancer is the first nursing intervention required for men with prostate cancer. These changes include: changes in potency among prostate cancer patients, including painful ejaculation, permanent reduction in semen volume, and decreased libido or sex drive. The major side effect is gradual and permanent loss of erectile function during the first year of treatment, and is probably caused by pelvic artery fibrosis, which has been researched by many (Schover, von Eschenbach, Smith, & Gonzalez, 1984; Litwin et al., 1999). Teaching and reassurance by the nurse that these changes are part of their disease allows men to understand their bodies and feel comfortable learning how to compensate for these disease-related changes.

An advantage of brachytherapy has been the high rate of preservation of sexual function as compared to external beam radiation and radical prostatectomy. Prostate brachytherapy is thought to have the lowest incidence of sexual dysfunction when compared to all the available treatment modalities (Benoit, Naslund, & Cohen, 2000). Within the implant population, it has been reported that 85% of men under 70 years of age were able to maintain potency after treatment and for those 70 years and older or those that had partial potency, they maintained an erection 47% of the time.

Common problems associated with potency include temporary burning with ejaculation, which is related to inflammation of ejaculatory ducts or the urethra due to radiation and painful ejaculation. Also, the amount of ejaculate may decrease in the months to years following implant therapy. Dry ejaculate or orgasm can occur in about 25% of implant patients. Hematospermia, which is blood in the semen, can occur intermittently after implant for many years (Blasko & Wallner, 1997).

The assessment of sexual dysfunction includes a thorough medical and psychiatric history, current medication profile, but most importantly, information regarding sexual function. This includes ability to have an erection, quality of erection, ability to maintain the erection for penetration, presence of nocturnal erections, ability to ejaculate, or decreased sexual drive or libido. A common tool used in the assessment of sexual dysfunction is the PLISSIT model. It is an acronym for permission, limited information, specific suggestions and intensive therapy. It focuses on giving patient permission to have sexual feelings, provides information, offers suggestions or recommendations and provides guidance in seeking assistance for specific interventions (Annon, 1974).

Patient teaching regarding the impact of prostate cancer and disease treatment is a primary nursing responsibility. The patients should be assured that their symptoms are manageable and should be instructed on the treatment options available. Following the assessment of sexual dysfunction, the treatment of sexual dysfunction includes medical and psychological interventions. First line therapy includes the use of oral erectogenic agents, most commonly known as Viagra® (sildenafil), vacuum constriction devices, and psychosexual counseling (Padma-Nathan & Forrest, 2000). Viagra® enhances the relaxant effect of nitric oxide released during sexual stimulation by increasing cyclic guanosine monophosphate (cGMP) in the corporal smooth muscle. This causes smooth muscle relaxation and increased arterial blood flow and corporal veno-occlusion, leading to an erection. The most common side effects are headaches, nasal congestion, flushing, and dyspepsia. Viagra® is contraindicated for patients taking nitrates in any form, such as Imdur® (isosorbide) and nitroglycerin, because it enhances cardiac preload reduction and the occurrence of hypotension, which can lead to myocardial infarction and cardiac arrest. The recommended dose is 50–100 mg taken one hour prior to sexual activity, with peak effect within two hours. Viagra® has no effect on libido. Merrick and colleagues (1999) have reported that Viagra® was effective in 80.6% of patients after brachytherapy and far more effective with patients who have undergone radical prostatectomy.

The vacuum constriction device (VCD) is another intervention, which is available for men who choose or have a contraindication to taking oral medications or participating in psychosexual counseling. The vacuum applies negative pressure to the non-erect penis and then draws venous blood flow into the penis. The erection is maintained by the use of an elastic band and will last for 20 to 30 minutes. Side effects associated with this method are penile pain, numbness, bruising, discolored penis (i.e., blue), and slowed ejaculation. Caution should be taken in men on anticoagulants, such as Coumadin® (warfarin sodium) due to increased bruisability.

Psychosexual therapy is another intervention available to men with prostate cancer and their partners. Sexual dysfunction can be accompanied by depression, decreased self-esteem and decreased satisfaction with relationships. The goal of sex therapy is to assist patients in accepting limitations and teach them to reduce anxiety and foster adaptation to a "new normal" sexual life. Sexual counseling focuses on the need for relaxation and a shift of focus from performance to pleasure. Couples need to explore the meaning of intimacy, which takes on many different forms.

Second-line interventions are utilized when patients fail first-line therapy or experience adverse reactions. These include intracavernosal injections of alprostadil, phentolamine or yohimbine and intraurethral administration of alprostadil, which are prostaglandins (Padma-Nathan & Forrest, 2000). Prostaglandins relax vascular smooth muscle by increasing cGMP, leading to an erection. With intracavernosal administration, the man or his partner can inject prostaglandin into the lateral aspect of the corpora cavernosum, using a 27- to 30-gauge needle. Onset of action is usually within 10 minutes and erection peaks at 30 to 60 minutes. Side effects of therapy include prolonged erections or priapism, penile pain, and scar tissue formation with prolonged use. It is recommended that no more than three injections per week be administered and not within a 24-hour period.

Intraurethral alprostadil (MUSE®) is another pharmacologic intervention in the treatment of erectile dysfunction. Its mechanism of action is the same as for intracavernosal injections. MUSE® is a suppository that is inserted into the urethra. The most common side effects include penile pain, feeling of warmth or burning in urethra, penis and groin, and redness of penis. Onset of action is within 5 to 10 minutes, with duration about 30 to 60 minutes. It should not be administered more than twice per day.

Third-line intervention for erectile dysfunction is surgical in nature. The implantation of semi-rigid or inflatable penile prostheses is utilized for those men with severe refractory erectile dysfunction. Most common complications include infection and skin erosion (Padma-Nathan & Forrest, 2000).

As nurses, it is important to be knowledgeable about the various interventions available in the treatment of sexual dysfunction and to feel comfortable in the delivery of our conversation, due to its delicate and intimate nature. In essence, health care professionals need to feel comfortable about their own sexuality. There are many available resources available for patients and their partners. One such resource is a support group for men with prostate cancer to assist them in exploring the issues of sexuality and intimacy. The American Cancer Society also offers a support service to men with prostate cancer called *Man to Man*. It provides men with the opportunity to talk about issues related to their cancer with other survivors of prostate cancer. They also provide an educational booklet called *Sexuality and Cancer: For the Man who has Cancer, and his Partner,* which may be beneficial. As mentioned earlier, referring couples to a sex therapist to explore and minimize anxieties about sexual dysfunction is extremely important.

PSYCHOSOCIAL ISSUES IN MEN WITH PROSTATE CANCER

The suspected and confirmed diagnosis of prostate cancer is a major stressful event that affects the patient and significant others. The diagnosis of cancer engenders feelings of hopelessness, sadness, guilt, frustration, alienation and vulnerability. Interventions to minimize distress and enhance the patient and family's ability to cope are critical during all phases of the cancer experience (Holmes, 1987). As health care professionals, we need to assist the patient to adapt and cope effectively with the experiences along the cancer journey.

Assessment includes the patient's preexisting coping skills, perceived meaning of the illness, anticipated loss of control over physical functioning, and the availability of family supports (Holmes, 1987). To guide the patient in maintaining or achieving psychosocial health, the factors that might affect adaptation must be identified. Previous experiences with crisis situations, perception of illness, coping mechanisms, and preparation of patient and family are essential factors in the patient's adjustment. Social support is another critical variable in the ongoing adaptation to the cancer experience. Patients must deal with the diagnosis, treatment effects, and uncertainty of the disease. Cancer patients can be emotionally devastated by the illness, particularly if little or no support is available. The uncertainties and fears experienced by a person diagnosed with cancer are likely to result in an enhanced need for social support. As patients contend with anxieties about pain, physical changes, treatment and recurrence, the need for support may intensify (Wortman, 1984). There are many sources of support from which prostate cancer patients can choose. They include spouse or significant others, family members, friends, neighbors, co-workers, pastoral care workers, health care professionals such as physicians, nurses, social workers, and those specializing in psychology or psychiatry, and lastly self-help or professional support groups.

Support groups are a complementary method of assisting patients and their families to face issues and overcome difficult, overwhelming situations. They provide excellent opportunities for learning, and there is evidence to suggest that when people are undergoing extreme distress, those who have similar experiences may be in a unique position to provide effective support (Wortman, 1984). This also is referred to as the "same boat" syndrome. There are four basic assumptions to support why cancer patients decide to attend support groups. They include verbalization of feelings, reception of empathy from others, seeking information about available resources, and informational needs about disease and treatment (Brown & Griffiths, 1986; Krizek, Roberts, Ragan, Ferrara, & Lord, 1999).

Support groups designed for men with prostate cancer assist in providing information to patients and their families regarding the disease process, treatment options, side effects of treatment, and self-care strategies. Most important, support groups provide a safe haven for men to verbalize feelings of impaired body image, sexual inadequacy, and issues centered on depression, anxiety, and fears of recurrence and death. Support groups are not the answer for all patients, but they have been found to be helpful for those who attend. Support groups guide patients in problem solving, decision making, instillation of hope, and verbalization of intimate feelings and emotions. As mentioned earlier, the American Cancer Society offers a support service to men with prostate cancer called *Man to Man*. The goals of the *Man to Man* program are to provide men with information about the diagnosis and treatment of prostate cancer, provide the support and encouragement to cope and solve common problems associated with the disease and to promote awareness of prostate cancer within the community (Coreil & Behal, 1999).

Spiegel, Bloom, and Yalom (1981) found that group members serve as role models for each other and depend on each other. Participation in a group with others who have the same life-threatening condition provides a sense of community and ameliorates the deep sense of isolation commonly experienced by cancer patients. The purpose of support groups is that sympathetic and direct confrontation with life and death issues results in mastery rather than demoralization. The group setting provides emotional support, enhances the patient's compilation of coping strategies, and diminishes the sense of isolation, helplessness and worthlessness. Spiegel (1990) researched women with metastatic breast cancer who attended or never attended a support group. He found that those women who attended a support group lived a mean of 18 months longer than those who never attended a support group. The reason these patients lived longer is unclear. However, he felt it was due to enhanced effectiveness of treatment along with decreased depression, increased appetite, decreased pain and discomfort and maintaining normal activity and lifestyle. Replication of such a study has not been done in the prostate cancer population. But Fawzy et al. (1993) has replicated it in the melanoma population with similar results. Gregoire, Kalogeropoulos, and Corcos (1997) investigated the effectiveness of a professionally facilitated prostate cancer support group and found encouraging results. They concluded that participants had a better understanding of their disease and felt more involved in their care. They also reported that patients had a sense of reassurance when sharing experiences related to prostate cancer, had decreased anxiety and had a more positive outlook.

The assessment and management of psychosocial issues must never be overlooked in the prostate cancer population. Whether patients choose to attend a support group or referrals for individual therapy are made, they have proven to be very helpful. These referral sources include oncology social workers, clinical psychologists, psychiatric advanced practice registered nurses (APRN), or psychiatrists.

In addition to dealing with side effects of treatment and disease and learning to cope with cancer, patients must deal with the associated anxiety that may surface before follow-up appointments and awaiting PSA results. The impact of prostate cancer is an emotional and physical rollercoaster with a plethora of emotions that evolve. The prostate cancer experience is unique in that patients cope very differently and that each situation is also very unique and individual. As health care professionals, it is important to recognize this and manage each patient in a specialized way that is appropriate for their situation, considering their values and belief system.

11
End of Life Care

Susan Derby and Diane B. Loseth

Cancer of the prostate is a devastating illness. At the time of diagnosis, many patients with prostate cancer are not eligible for curative treatment. The treatment of prostate cancer varies with stage of disease. Treatment choices for Stages I and II are generally managed by radical surgery and radiation therapy. Locally advanced tumors are generally treated with external beam radiation therapy, alone or in combination with androgen ablation. Complications of radical prostatectomy include impotence, the inability to have or maintain an erection which may occur in upwards of 98% of patients (Stock, 1995). Early complications from radiation therapy are cystitis, proctitis and diarrhea. Treatment decisions are generally based on the patient's age, life expectancy, potential side effect profile of treatment and impact on the patient's quality of life. All forms of treatment are associated with about a 10-year survival (Chodak, 1994; Stock, 1995). The main indicator of shorter survival is poorly differentiated disease—Gleason score ≥ 7, (Chodak et al., 1994), although other predictors of relapse include clinical stage 2b or greater, and Prostate-specific antigen (PSA) over 25 ng/ml.

Advanced prostate cancer is conventionally treated with hormonal therapy. Prostate cancer is under the influence of androgen hormones; androgen deprivation can produce regression of disease and improvement in symptoms and quality of life. For patients whose disease is refractory to hormone therapy, chemotherapy, namely, mitoxantrone is an option.(Tannock et al., 1996). The median survival for men whose metastatic disease is refractory to hormonal treatment, is one year.

When patients develop metastatic disease one of the goals is symptom management. End of life care involves management of symptoms with a focus on the quality of life. Progressive, metastatic prostate cancer is associated with a host of symptoms that contribute to the death of the patient. Numerous studies have evaluated symptoms during the last weeks of life and indicate that patients experience a high degree of symptom distress and suffering (Fainsinger et al., 1991; Ng & von Guten, 1998; Ventafridda et al., 1990). Studies have shown that the most prevalent and difficult symptoms to manage in dying patients are pain, dyspnea, and confusional states (Fainsinger et al., 1991; Ventafridda et al., 1990). Other symptoms include fatigue, anemia, lymphedema, hydronephrosis, anxiety, and depression (Esper & Redman, 1999; Krishnasamy, 2000; Colombel, Mallame, & Abbou, 1997; Payne & Massie, 2000; Pilepich, Asbell, Mulholland, & Pajak, 1984; Piper et al., 1991; Wilson, Chochinov, deFaye, & Breitbart, 2000).

The complex symptomatology experienced by patients with prostate cancer demands an aggressive approach to symptom assessment and intervention. Devising an end of life plan of care requires symptom assessment, ongoing communication with the patient and family, and understanding of the goals of care. Dimensions of an end of life care plan for the patient with prostate cancer are outlined in Table 11.1. This chapter presents the major symptoms commonly experienced with prostate cancer at the end of life and management of those symptoms. Issues related to caregivers and psychological distress, as it effects the patient and their caregiver, will be discussed.

PAIN

Patients with advanced disease may develop either nociceptive or neuropathic pain syndromes. Nociceptive pain may be due to intraabdominal/pelvic or bony disease. Neuropathic pain may be due to compression or infiltration of nerves. Adenocarcinoma of the prostate spreads most commonly to the well-vascularized areas of the skeleton, including the spine, ribs, skull, and proximal end of the long bones. The mechanism of metasasis is via Batson's plexus, a low pressure, high volume system of vertebral veins which ascends the spine.

Bone metastases are a catastrophic occurrence for many patients, often interfering with the function and quality of life. Pain is often the primary symptom, occurring in up to 62% of patients at diagnosis (Tofe, Francis, & Harvey, 1975), and in 50% to 75% of patients with advanced disease (Galasko, 1982). Metastatic bone disease frequently causes morbidity, spinal cord compression, and pathological fractures. Bone metastases usually produce pain and decreased quality of life. Pathologic fractures occurring spontaneously or following injury are common and

TABLE 11.1 Dimensions of an End of Life Care Plan for the Patient with Prostate Cancer

Assess extent of disease documented by imaging studies and laboratory data.

Assess symptoms including prevalence, severity and impact on function.

Aggressively manage most distressing symptoms identified by the patient.

Identify coping strategies and psychological symptoms including presence of anxiety, depression and suicidality.

Evaluate religious and spiritual beliefs.

Assess over-all quality of life and well-being—does the patient feel secure that all that can be done for them is being done? Is the patient satisfied with the present level of symptom control?

Determine family burden—Is attention being paid to the caregiver so that burnout does not occur? If the spouse or caregiver is elderly, are they able to meet the physical demands of caring for the patient?

Determine level of care needed in the home.

Assess financial burden on patient and caregiver—Is an inordinate amount of money being spent on patient and will there be adequate provisions for the caregiver when the patient dies?

Identify presence of advance care planning requests—Have the patient's wishes and preferences for resuscitation, artificial feeding and hydration been discussed? Has the patient identified a surrogate decision-maker who knows his/her wishes? Is there documentation regarding advance directives?

---

occur more frequently in patients with osteolytic disease. They occur most frequently in the vertebral bodies and the proximal ends of long bones, both common sites of metastatic disease (Mundy, 1997).

Fractures involving the proximal femur are the most common surgical issue in the management of bone metastases. Normal activity, such as walking, rising from a chair, climbing stairs, or lifting the leg to get in or out of bed, applies forces exceeding three times a person's body weight to the hip and the proximal femur (Healey & Brown, 1997). Any underlying mechanical weakness due to metastatic disease can easily result in fracture.

The most common presenting symptom for epidural cord compression is back pain. Spinal cord compression may occur when tumors invade and impinge directly on the spinal cord. More frequently, however, severe, destructive osteolytic lesions lead to fracture and fragility of one or more of the vertebral bodies (Mundy, 1997). In addition, other symptoms such as bowel and/or bladder dysfunction, or leg weakness may be present.

Nerve compression syndromes also occur in patients with osteoblastic lesions because of bony overgrowths that impinge directly on spinal nerves. Another site of nerve compression is the cauda equina. In addition, cranial nerve involvement from base of skull disease may occur.

Assessment

Initial and ongoing assessment of pain should include attention to intensity, location, pain descriptors, timing, duration, and aggravating or alleviating factors. Patients with prostate cancer often have multiple sites of pain, and all sites need to be assessed. Patients with bone pain usually describe it as dull and intermittent, aggravated by movement, weight-bearing or both. Bone pain is most commonly characterized by its incidental nature and may be episodic, related to increased activity such as ambulation or a change in position. Patients may report local bone tenderness and worsening pain at night.

Assessment of pain for men with prostate cancer is an essential part of pain management. There are many standardized tools for objectively assessing pain in older adults. Some patients find categorical scales using words easier to use than numbers (0–10). Subsequent pain assessment should consistently use the same tool, realizing that as patients become more ill, numerical rating scales may be replaced by words, or nonverbal assessments. Several pain instruments are summarized in Table 11.2, along with their advantages and disadvantages.

Barriers to Cancer Pain Management

Barriers to cancer pain management have been well described in the literature (AHCPR, 1994; Joransen, Cleeland, Weissman, & Gilson, 1992; McCaffery & Ferrell, 1992a, b, c, 1993; Von Roenn et al., 1993). Undertreatment of pain is a consequence of these barriers. The barriers can be divided into patient/family, provider, and regulatory barriers. Patients and families are concerned about addiction, tolerance, and side effects of pain medications. Another fear is that pain signals progression of the cancer.

Health care providers express some of the same concerns (Von Roenn et al., 1993). Lack of knowledge is the most common reason for these fears and misconceptions. As a consequence, assessment and management is poor. McCaffery and Ferrell (1991, 1992a, b, c) found that nurses were less likely to give adequate doses of pain medications to those who were older, who had a nonconformist lifestyle, were female, and who had

TABLE 11.2 Pain Assessment Instruments and Major Advantages and Disadvantages

Assessment Instruments	Major Advantages	Major Disadvantages
Numeric Rating Scale (NRS)	Patients are simply asked to rate their pain on an abstract scale of 0–10	The abstract design of the scale makes it difficult for some older adults to understand, especially the cognitively impaired population.
Visual Analogue Scales (VAS) (Carlsson, 1983)	Easy to administer to most patients, including those who are cognitively impaired, or who have language, hearing and speech deficits. Good reliability and validity.	The inconvenience of administering these paper and pencil scales may preclude use in fast-paced clinical environments.
The McGill Pain Questionnaire (MPQ) (Melzack, & Katz, 1992)	The present pain inventory (PPI) and verbal description (VDS) subscales of the MPQ are effective apart from the entire MPQ. The tool is reliable with cognitively intact, cognitively impaired and community-based.	Lengthy instrument that requires completion of paper and pencil scale. Patients with visual and hearing impairments have difficulty understanding the entire questionnaire and become tired during the assessment.

Note. Adapted from Wallace, M. (2001). Pain Assessment Instruments. *Encyclopedia of Care for the Elderly*, New York: Springer Publishing.

minor alterations in vital signs. Follow-up studies (McCaffery & Ferrell, 1997) indicate that nurses' knowledge base has increased (higher percentage of correct answers) since those earlier studies, but there are still considerable deficits in accepting patients' self-report, increasing an opioid dose and addiction. In the interim, federal guidelines have been published (Jacox et al., 1994). Another impetus for change is the new pain standards of the Joint Commission on the Accreditation of Healthcare Organizations.

Educational programs addressing these barriers have been developed. The most well known is the Role Model Program (Weissman, Dahl, & Beasley, 1993) originated by the Wisconsin Cancer Pain Initiative. This program pairs health care professionals either in nurse-physician, nurse-pharmacist, or pharmacist-physician dyads. The goal is to select individuals from multiple organizations who have the ability to effect change in their own institution. In addition, several institutions have described methods to change attitudes, knowledge, and practices in their facility (Bookbinder et al., 1996; Ferrell et al., 1993). There are a wealth of resources available to the clinician to improve cancer pain management (Gordon, Dahl, & Stevenson, 1996; Pasero 1999; American Alliance of Cancer Pain Initiatives).

Opioids

Opioids continue to be the mainstay of cancer pain management. The World Health Organization in 1996 recommended a rationale for therapy for cancer pain based on assessment of intensity. (World Health Organization, 1996). For moderate to severe pain, higher doses of opioids with or without an adjuvant or non-opioid are recommended. The National Comprehensive Cancer Network (2001), the Agency for Health Care Policy and Research (Jacaox et al., 1994), and the American Pain Society (1999) have recommended the use of opioids for cancer pain.

When selecting an opioid, one needs to consider the renal clearance of the patient. Patients with prostate cancer often have co-morbid conditions or are at an advanced age. These two factors place them at greater risk for potential side effects of opioids due to illness and age-related alterations in pharmacokinetics, specifically distribution and elimination. In the elderly patient with prostate cancer, there may be an age-related change in renal function which may impact upon opioid management. The effect of age on renal function is variable; some studies show a linear decrease in renal function, other studies show no change in creatinine clearance with advancing age (Vestal, 1997). Renal mass decreases 25% to 30% in advanced age and renal blood flow decreases 1% per year after age 50 (Vestal, 1997). As a result, the metabolite of morphine, morphine-6 glucuronide, may accumulate with repeated dosing, especially in the setting of impaired renal or hepatic function in the elderly patient with prostate cancer (Sjogren, 1997). This may mean that morphine is not the most suitable opioid in the prostate cancer patient with impaired renal function. If, after several days of treatment with morphine, the patient develops side effects such as sedation or confusion, it may mean that there is an accumulation of these metabolites. It is therefore reasonable to change the opioid. At the same time, other potential causes of the side effects should be investigated, such as metabolic changes or infection.

Meperidine is not recommended for chronic use in the cancer population. With repeated dosing of meperidine, there may be delayed renal excretion of meperidine's metabolite normeperidine. This may result in delirium, central nervous system stimulation, myoclonus, and seizures.

Long-acting opioids, such as controlled-release morphine, oxycodone, and the fentanyl patch minimize the number of doses the patient must take. Minimizing the number of doses allows for ease of administration. With close monitoring, opioids with longer half-lives such as methadone can be safely used. Table 11.3 outlines the most commonly used opioids in the prostate cancer patient at the end of life. Parenteral routes of administration should be considered in patients who require rapid onset of analgesia, or who require high doses of opioids that cannot be administered orally. They may be administered in a variety of ways including the intravenous and subcutaneous route using a patient controlled analgesia (PCA) device.

Patients who are dying are particularly susceptible to opioid-induced constipation, and a laxative and stool softener should be prescribed (Derby & Portenoy, 1997). The initial presentation of constipation can be confusing and, in most cases, multifactorial. Abdominal signs and symptoms including pain, distension, and nausea may be absent. The patient may present with confusion, depressed mood, and loss of appetite. Assessment of medications should include all medications, including those with anticholinergic properties, and over-the-counter medications such as iron preparations and antacids. At the end of life, when the goals of care are comfort, it is vitally important to maintain bowel function through use of oral laxatives, and when that is no longer possible, with suppositories or enemas. Constipation can be a source of severe pain and suffering and should always be aggressively managed. If left untreated, it seriously affects the quality of life of the patient.

Adjuvants

Steroids and nonsteroidal anti-inflammatory agents (NSAIDs) are especially useful in the management of bone pain and inflammation. When used concurrently with opioids, lower doses of opioids may be an additional

TABLE 11.3 Common Opioids Used at the End of Life in Patients With Prostate Cancer

Opioid	Comments
Morphine	Observe for side effects with repeated dosing
Hydromorphone	Short half-life opioid, may be safer than morphine
Propoxyphene (Darvon, Darvocet)	Avoid use, metabolite causes CNS and cardiac toxicity
Codeine	May cause severe constipation, nausea/vomiting
Methadone	Use carefully, long half-life may produce side effects. Monitor carefully during first 72 hours of initiation. Use a short-acting opioid as needed
Transdermal Fentanyl Patch	Cannot titrate easily, use only if stable pain
Demerol	Avoid in chronic pain patients due to CNS toxicity
Oxycodone	Useful, especially long-acting preparation and when patients cannot tolerate morphine

benefit. Short-term use of steroids is generally safe and effective, and their use should be considered as an effective palliative care measure during the last weeks and months of life.

There are some well-known side effects of NSAIDs. Elderly patients with a history of ulcer disease are most vulnerable to the gastrointestinal side effects of these drugs (Wolfe, Lichtenstein, & Singh, 1999). They can also cause renal insufficiency and nephrotoxicity and are problematic in patients with congestive heart failure or peripheral edema. Cognitive dysfunction has been reported with the use of salicylates, indomethacin, naproxen, and ibuprofen (Egbert, 1996; Moore & O'Keefe, 1999; Roth, 1989) Evaluation of the risk versus benefit ratio to the patient is important, and at the end of life, the benefit of NSAIDs may outweigh the risk. A new class of NSAIDs selectively blocks the cyclooxygenase-2 (COX-2) enzymatic pathway, which is induced by tissue injury or other inflammation-inducing conditions. There appears to be less risk of gastrointestinal bleeding, renal dysfunction, and generalized bleeding with prolonged use of the COX-2 agents (Cryer & Feldman 1998).

For patients with neuropathic pain syndromes—for example, lumbosacral plexopathy—other adjuvants may be beneficial. The adjuvants used for neuropathic pain are, most commonly, antidepressants and anticonvulsants. As with opioids, these drugs require monitoring and titration for effect.

Pharmacological Considerations

The major focus of nursing management of pain and other symptoms of the dying patient with prostate cancer is pharmacological treatment. The use of multiple medications, or polypharmacy, may contribute to worsening side effects. If, for example, the patient is experiencing sedation from the opioid and has good pain control, with rare rescue use, it may be acceptable to decrease the 24-hour total dose. Another strategy is to add a psychostimulant, such as methylphenidate or dextroamphetamine daily or twice a day, which will counter the sedation. Psychostimulants often work quickly. Patients on psychostimulants should be assessed for irritability, tremors, anxiety, and insomnia. Changing the opioid can be another strategy to minimize or treat side effects. A careful medication review should always be done prior to the initiation of a new drug.

Radiotherapy, Bisphosphonates, and Radioisotopes

Prostate carcinoma frequently metastasizes to the skeleton, causing significant morbidity, including bone pain, pathological fractures, epidural cord compression, and hypercalcemia. More than 50% of patients with prostate cancer will develop bone metastases (Garfunkel, 1991). Malignant infiltration into bone produces osteoclast stimulation which is responsible for bone destruction (osteoclysis) and subsequent bone resorption. In metastatic bone disease there is a net loss of bone (Galasko, 1982; Pereira, Mancini, & Walker, 1998).

When there is osteoblastic disease, as in prostate cancer, there is increased bone density due to the formation of new bone around the tumor. Osteoblasts are bone-forming cells in the bone marrow. The incidence of pure osteoblastic metastases is 95% for metastatic prostate cancer (Adami, 1997). It has become increasingly clear that even when there are osteoblastic sites of disease, there is an increase in bone resorption as well.

Tumor cells frequently metastasize to the most heavily vascularized part of bone, particularly the red bone marrow of the axial skeleton and the proximal ends of the long bones, the ribs, and the vertebral column. The management of bone metastases represents an effort to restore function and relieve pain. Treatment includes the use of analgesics, radiotherapy, bisphosphonates, and radioisotopes.

Radiation therapy (RT) is the most common treatment for painful bone lesions. Factors considered prior to initiating RT are previous radiation, including total dosage and location of previous RT, and bone marrow compromise. Bone metastases are generally treated with shorter radiation courses that deliver a lower total dose but give a higher dose with each treatment. In one study of radiotherapy for painful bone metastases, 205 patients were treated with conventional fractionation (40–46 Gy in 20–23 fractions over 5–5.5 weeks), short course (30–36 Gy in 10–12 fractions over 2–2.3 weeks), or fast course (8–28 Gy in 1–4 consecutive fractions). Eighty-three percent of those patients with prostate cancer obtained complete pain relief (Arcangeli et al., 1998). For patients who have a limited life expectancy, shorter courses of radiation therapy may be considered.

Bisphosphonates have been demonstrated to reduce the incidence of fracture and reduce the severity of pain from painful bone metastases (Ernst, 1998; Pereira, Mancini, & Walker, 1998). Analogs of pyrophosphate, bisphosphonates, are absorbed into mineralized bone after systemic administration. Bisphosphonates (etidronate, clodronate, pamidronate) are drugs that stabilize bone minerals, thus inhibiting bone resorption. The most commonly used bisphosphonate is pamidronate. Twenty-five to forty percent of intravenously administered doses are excreted by the kidneys. The remainder is absorbed by bone. Pain relief may take days to weeks. Therefore, one must consider the life expectancy of the patient and the benefit versus burden of administering this drug. Side effects that may occur are flu-like symptoms, ocular complications, or exacerbation of pain.

In a randomized, nonblinded study of 42 prostate cancer patients who received weekly 30 mg dose of intravenous pamidronate, 44% reported a decrease in reported pain (Clarke, McClure, & George, 1992). Other studies in patients with breast cancer (Hortobagyi et al., 1996) and multiple myeloma (Berenson et al., 1996) found decreases in mean baseline pain scores. Presently, many clinicians recommend administering pamidronate 60 mg to 90 mg intravenously every 3 to 4 weeks to patients with painful bone disease (Fulfaro, Casuccio, Ticozzi, & Ripamonti, 1998).

The use of pamidronate to manage painful blastic lesions has not been adequately demonstrated, although there is evidence that there is bone resorption with osteoblastic metastases (Adami, 1997). However, many clinicians are administering it because the side effects are minimal, and it is well tolerated. In a review of the literature on the development of evidence-based guidelines in palliative care, Mannix and colleagues (2000) reported that: a) overall, studies demonstrate efficacy of bisphosphonates in patients with breast cancer and multiple myeloma; and b) 50% to 60% of patients (with blastic or lytic lesions) with a variety of malignancies respond within 14 days, and therefore, a response may be obtained in some patients with prostate cancer. Based on this review, the authors of this study recommended the use of bisphosphonates in patients with any diagnosis, when treatment with conventional analgesics, radiotherapy, or orthopedic surgery is unsuccessful or inappropriate.

Bone-seeking radioisotopes have been used in the management of bone pain. The indications for use of radioisotopes are poorly controlled pain from multiple, bony sites. The two most common radioisotopes are Strontium-89 and Samarium-153. These isotopes are absorbed at the site of osteoclastic activity and are therefore best used in patients with osteoblastic lesions, including patients with prostate cancer (Serafini, 1994). One advantage of Samarium is that bone scans can be used to monitor its effect on bony sites of disease. Studies of radioisotopes in patients with prostate cancer have shown to be equally effective as conventional radiation in the management of pain (Brudage, Crook, & Lukka, 1998; Serafini et al., 1998). Strontium-89 may preclude further systemic chemotherapy due to bone marrow suppression (Brudage et al., 1998), but this is not usually an issue at the end of life. Studies have found a reduction of pain in up to 60% to 90% of patients (Laing et al., 1991; Lewington et al., 1991; Porter et al., 1993; Quilty et al., 1994). The most common side effect is a transient increase in pain lasting 36 to 48 hours, occurring 1 to 2 weeks after initiation of therapy (Nightengale et al., 1995). In most cases, pain relief begins within one week, but may occur earlier with Samarium. Patients must have an adequate bone marrow reserve and no evidence of spinal cord compression (Serafini et al., 1998; Quilty, et al., 1994).

Surgical Approaches in the Management of Cancer Pain

Anesthetic and neurosurgical approaches are indicated when conservative measures utilizing opioids and adjuvant analgesics have failed to provide adequate analgesia or when the patient is experiencing intolerable side effects of analgesics such as sedation or nausea and vomiting. At the end of life, one should evaluate the impact of hospitalization and morbidity associated with aggressive interventional procedures. The clearest indication for these approaches is the patient who is unable to benefit from systemic pharmacological approaches to pain management because of intolerable toxicity. These procedures include regional analgesia (spinal, intraventricular, and intrapleural opioids), sympathetic blockade and neurolytic procedures (celiac plexus block, lumbar sympathetic block, cervicothoracic [stellate] ganglion block), or pathway ablation procedure (chemical or surgical rhizotomy, or cordotomy). For patients requiring orthopedic intervention to repair or stabilize a fracture (e.g., humerus, vertebral body), quality of life issues, discussed in chapter 5, and life expectancy, need to be considered.

Nonpharmacological Approaches: Complementary Therapies

Complementary therapies, such as cognitive-behavioral interventions, relaxation, guided imagery, distraction, and music therapy, can be used as an adjunct to pharmacological and surgical approaches to manage pain in the prostate cancer patient. These approaches carry few side effects and, when possible, should be tried along with other approaches. The major advantages of these techniques are that they are easy to learn, safe and often readily accepted by patients. Cognitive and behavioral interventions may be helpful in reducing emotional distress, improving coping, and offering the patient and family a sense of control. In selecting an approach, factors that should be considered include physical and psychological burden to the patient, efficacy, and practicality. These strategies may offer the patient a reduction in systemic analgesic use thereby diminishing adverse effects. In one study of 60 prostate cancer patients, 80% reported trying at least one complementary/alternative medicine since being diagnosed with prostate cancer. The most widely used modality was nutritional supplements, followed by dietary modification, herbal treatments, and meditation (Jacobson, Grann, & Neugut, 1999).

FATIGUE

Fatigue is one of the most pervasive symptoms among cancer patients. Cancer-related fatigue might be defined as a clinical syndrome characterized by generalized weakness and both physical and mental exhaustion (Bruera & MacDonald, 1988). Studies have documented fatigue as a major symptom at the end of life (Coyle, Adelhardt, Foley, & Portenoy, 1990; Krishnasamy, 2000). The etiology of fatigue in cancer patients is often multifactorial. In patients with prostate cancer at the end of life, causes such as pain, extent of disease, recent radiation therapy, or chemotherapy, anemia, dyspnea, and depression may be significant contributors to fatigue. Interventions used to manage or prevent fatigue are dependent upon the etiology. The interventions are divided into active exercise, attention, restoration, preparatory education, and psychosocial education

(Dean & Anderson, 2001). If, for example, the fatigue is related to uncontrolled pain or dyspnea, or to anemia, aggressive management of those symptoms should be done. Regardless of the etiology, establishing a regular bedtime and awakening schedule, provision for rest periods throughout the day, pharmacologic management of insomnia, if present, and use of behavioral approaches may be helpful. For a further discussion of fatigue see chapter 7.

ANEMIA

Harrison (2000) retrospectively examined the records of 202 radiation therapy patients with a variety of tumor types. Men with prostate cancer had a 32% incidence of anemia during radiation therapy. The adverse effects of anemia extend beyond course of radiation therapy. Anemia can also cause exertional dyspnea, dizziness, vertigo, palpitations, tachycardia, systolic ejection murmur, congestive heart failure, depression, anorexia, nausea, cognitive impairment, insomnia, indigestion and lowered body temperature (Harrison, 2000). Therefore, attempts to correct symptomatic anemia and its negative sequela should be undertaken. The judicious use of transfusions may significantly improve the quality of life. In patients who cannot tolerate transfusions, or in whom transfusions are inappropriate, the administration of recombinant human erythropoietin may be indicated, when appropriate.

LYMPHEDEMA

Lymphedema is the accumulation of large amounts of interstitial fluid caused by lymphatic obstruction. Although lymphedema may occur after RT to the pelvis or surgical manipulation of the lymphatics (e.g., staging lymphadenectomy) in patients with advanced prostate cancer, the lymphatic obstruction is commonly due to tumor infiltration (Petrek, Pressman, & Smith, 2000; Tunkel & Rampulla, 1998). The volume of lymphatic fluid exceeds the body's ability to circulate the fluid, resulting in edema and fibrosis in the extremities. This static fluid leads to an increased risk for infection, precipitating the development of cellulitis.

Studies on lymphedema have not included patients at the end of life. The Radiation Therapy Oncology Group (Pilepich, Asbell, Mulholland, & Pajak, 1984) reported 30% to 66% incidence of lymphedema in 136 prostate patients after staging lymphadenectomies. Other authors have reported that patients with lymphedema have noted severe limitations in physical function, depression and anxiety, as well as complaints of heaviness and pain (Carter, 1997; Newman, Brennan, & Passik, 1996; Passik, Newman, Brennan, & Holland, 1993). In patients with prostate cancer, lymphedema generally begins in the distal part of the leg and gradually increases up the lower extremity into the thighs, lower pelvis, and scrotum. Lymphedema can be unilateral or bilateral. At the end of life, as the tumor in the lower pelvis increases, leg swelling can become severe, making ambulating and even moving the limb, quite distressing. While leg wrapping and gradient pressure treatments have been somewhat successful in treating lymphedema, patients at the end of life are often too debilitated to participate in such treatments.

HYDRONEPHROSIS

Hydronephrosis occurs when the pelvis and calices of one or both kidneys become dilated, causing an obstruction in the flow of urine (*Stedman's Medical Dictionary*, 1990). In the patient with prostate cancer, hydronephrosis is caused by local extension of the tumor and tumor spread along the lymphatics (Colombel, Mallame, & Abbou, 1997). As urinary obstruction and renal function deteriorates, patients commonly have percutaneous nephrostomy (PCN) tubes placed. This actually may extend their life expectancy by improvement of renal function. Studies showed survival rates in prostate cancer patients after PCN were 55% to 60% at one year (Bordinazzo, Benecchi, Cazzaniga, Vercesi, & Privitera, 1994; Chiou, Chang, & Horn, 1990). Pappas and colleagues (2000) evaluated the effectiveness of PCN tube placement. Of the 206 patients in the study, 125 had a malignancy. Two thirds of patients with urinary obstruction had renal function return to normal, but the patient population was mixed with malignant and benign urinary obstructions. Lack of renal improvement was associated with being older and having prostate cancer. In another study, survival in prostate cancer patients who had PCN tube(s) placed, was significantly worse in those who had failed hormone therapy. The mean survival was 80 days for those with progressive disease versus 646 days for those who had yet to receive hormonal treatment (Paul, Love, & Chisholm, 1994).

Having a PCN is not without an additional burden of care. Psychologically, patients have to adjust to having a stent(s) and coping with a urinary bag attached to them. Because PCNs are placed posteriorly, it requires the assistance of a caregiver to perform dressing changes and monitor the site for signs of infection. When patients are in the last one to two weeks of life, this burden of care is weighed into the decision to offer this procedure.

ANXIETY

Anxiety is frequently associated with medical illness. Uncontrolled symptoms, such as pain or dyspnea, side effects from medications (e.g., feeling jittery from steroids, akasthesia from phenothiazines) are examples of this type of anxiety. Metabolic causes and hormone producing tumors can also cause feelings of anxiety (Massie & Holland, 1992; Payne & Massie, 2000). When anxiety is suspected, the illness or symptoms related to the illness need to be treated before anxiolytics are initiated. For example, if a patient is experiencing dyspnea and anxiety, the anxiety may resolve once the dyspnea is controlled. The same holds true for other symptoms such as pain. A recent study of patients with cancer-related pain, with or without breakthrough pain, found that those with breakthrough pain had more anxiety than those without breakthrough pain (Portenoy, Payne, & Jacobsen, 1999). Knowledge of this fact may allow for earlier treatment of anxiety.

When the underlying cause(s) of the anxiety cannot be determined or alleviated, the most appropriate management is pharmacologic. Benzodiazepines are the most commonly used medications to treat anxiety. Administering these medications on an around-the-clock (ATC) schedule provides for more effective symptom control. Occasionally, anxiety can progress to severe agitation with or without delirium. When this occurs, a continuous infusion of a sedative may be helpful. Table 11.4 shows the most common anxiolytics used in the dying prostate cancer patient.

Anxious patients may also benefit from behavioral therapies such as guided imagery or relaxation techniques or other activities that decrease levels of anxiety. Psychotherapy at the end of life is not appropriate; however, counseling may be instrumental in helping patients at the end of

TABLE 11.4 Common Benzodiazepines Used in Dying Patients

Benzodiazepine	Usual Dosage	Comments
Lorazepam	0.25-2mg q4-6h	Short-acting; comes in several routes (po, SL, IV); may worsen a delirium
Clonazepam	0.25 qhs-1mg tid	Long-acting; only route is oral
Alprazolam	0.25-1mg tid	Effective in panic states; only route is oral

life resolve issues that are causing anxiety. Many patients at the end express concerns regarding dependency, financial worries, and role changes. Patients may also feel anxiety about their impending death, have a fear of the unknown, or may experience existential or spiritual distress (Payne & Massie, 2000).

In a review of the literature related to psychological interventions, Sellick and Crooks (1999) found that addressing psychological needs is indeed important, but no one method of assisting the patient and family is better than another. The drawback to this review was that none of the studies reviewed included patients at the end of life. Therefore, doing some of the simple things, such as providing a supportive environment, helping with practical matters, and assisting the patient in finding meaning in his illness and his dying are important interventions.

DEPRESSION

Studies investigating depression in the terminally ill are few. Yet, the available studies show that the prevalence rate increases up to 58% in patients at the end of life (Breitbart, Breura, Chochinov & Lynch, 1995; Chochinov, Wilson, Enns, & Lander, 1994; Wilson, Chochinov, de Faye, & Breitbart, 2000). One study examined the quality of life of prostate patients, comparing those undergoing various primary treatments. Twenty-one percent indicated feeling depressed (Kornblith, Herr, Ofman, Scher, & Holland, 1994). None of the patients in this study were at the end of their lives.

Depression may be related to poorly controlled symptoms. Ancedotally, symptoms that are undertreated or refractory to treatment, such as nausea, vomiting, and pain can cause a patient to be overwhelmed by the symptom and feel hopeless and helpless. Patients with severe pain may feel that life is unbearable and may express suicidal thoughts (Ciaramella & Poli, 2001). Once the pain is controlled, depression and suicidal ideation often subsides (Roth & Breitbart, 1996).

The DSM-IV criteria for depression are not especially useful when applied to the terminally ill because the symptoms that describe depression are frequently present in patients at the end of life. Insomnia, somnolence, anorexia, weight loss, fatigue, loss of energy, difficulty concentrating, and thoughts of death may naturally occur as cancer progresses and patients approach the end of their lives (Roth & Breitbart, 1996). Endicott (1984) identified four symptoms that represent the affect of dying patients. Those symptoms are depressed appearance, social withdrawal or decreased talkativeness, brooding or pessimism, and lack of reactivity. Roth and Breitbart (1996) have suggested that feelings of hopelessness, helplessness, worthlessness, guilt, and suicidal ideation are more indicative of depression in the terminally-ill patient. Another simple screening tool, a "distress thermometer," allows for easy assessment of depression. A group of prostate patients used this tool based on the visual analog scale that is used for pain. They rated their distress from 0 to 10 with word anchors of no distress at 0, moderate distress at 5, and extreme distress at 10. This global scale evaluated patients' emotional distress, though not specific to depression or anxiety. A score of ≥ 5 prompted a referral to the liaison for psychiatry in this study (Roth et al., 1998).

Physicians and nurses often fail to recognize depression in their patients (Hardman, Maguire, & Crowther, 1989; McDonald et al., 1999; Passik et al., 1998). Lack of knowledge, time constraints, fears of over medicating, adverse reactions and polypharmacy, and low priority all contribute to the underdiagnosis and undertreatment of depression (Block, 2000; Wilson, Chochinov, deFaye, & Breitbart, 2000). Antidepressants are most useful when life expectancy is several months. When death is expected within weeks, the use of psychostimulants, such as methylphenidate, may be the best choice. These medications have a short time to onset, and patients report increased energy and alertness within a day or few days (Roth & Breitbart, 1996; Wilson, Chochinov, deFaye, & Breitbart, 2000;).

Depression is not an inevitable part of dying. Even occasional thoughts of suicide are considered normal in the dying patient; however, an increased frequency of suicidal ideation needs further intervention. The dying person is losing everything and everyone in his life. Certainly sadness and feelings of loss are appropriate.

DELIRIUM

Delirium is a symptom that contributes significantly to increased morbidity and mortality. Estimates of the prevalence of delirium range from 25% to 40% in patients with cancer at some point during their disease. In the terminal phases of cancer the incidence increases to 85% (Breitbart et al., 1995; Foreman, 1993; Lipowski, 1990). Patients with delirium may exhibit mild confusion, hallucinations, agitation, or any combination of these symptoms. One of the major problems in the treatment of delirium is lack of assessment and intervention by hospital staff, especially if the patient is quiet and noncommunicative. Undertreatment of delirium results from the lack of assessment tools, inadequate knowledge of early signs of confusion, and inadequate time spent with the patient to determine cognitive function. In addition, behavioral manifestations include a variety of symptoms that may be interpreted as depression, psychosis or dementia. One tool that assesses the severity of delirium in medically ill patients is the 10-item Memorial Delirium Assessment Scale (MDAS). It evaluates cognitive functioning, psychomotor activity, and disturbances in arousal and level of consciousness (Breitbart et al., 1997).

The etiology of delirium in patients at the end of life is frequently multifactorial. Factors contributing to delirium are disease effects on the central nervous system, organ failure, electrolyte imbalance, infection, hypoxemia, hypothermia, hyperthermia, uncontrolled pain, sensory deprivation, sleep deprivation, medications, alcohol or drug withdrawal, constipation, or urinary retention. A variety of drugs can produce delirium in the prostate cancer patient (Table 11.5). In the palliative care setting, polypharmacy may be the only way to control symptoms at the end of life. To reduce the risk of polypharmacological induced delirium, it is prudent to add one medication at a time, evaluating its response, before adding another medication.

Treatment of delirium includes the identification of the underlying cause, correction of the precipitating factors, and symptom management of the delirium. At the end of life, the etiology may be multifactorial, and the cause is often irreversible. If delirium is occurring in the dying patient with prostate cancer, diagnostic evaluations (imaging and laboratory studies) may not be appropriate.

Pharmacologic treatment includes the use of sedatives and neuroleptics. Breitbart and Jacobsen (1996) have demonstrated that the use of lorazepam alone in controlling symptoms of delirium was ineffective and contributed to worsening cognition. They have advocated the use of a neuroleptic such as haloperidol along with a benzodiazepine in the control of an agitated delirium. All psychotropic drugs bind to plasma albumin and are excreted primarily by the kidney. Decreased serum albumin levels in the elderly, or those who have alterations in renal function, are at greater risk for toxic responses of these drugs (Salzman, 1991). The elderly may be more susceptible to the extrapyramidal side effects of antipsychotics, especially the akathisia, parkinsonism and akinesia (Salzman, 1991). Akathisia, or agitation, is often misdiagnosed as agitation. Akinesia, consisting of decreased speech and energy can often be misdiagnosed as depression. A newer neuroleptic, risperidone, has also been used to treat delirium and may have less side effects. The oral route is preferred, although in cases of severe agitation and delirium the parenteral route is more practical. Other interventions that may be helpful include restoration of fluid and electrolyte balance, environmental changes, and supportive techniques such as elimination of unnecessary stimuli, provision of a safe environment, and measures that reduce anxiety.

TABLE 11.5 Drugs Commonly Causing Delirium in the Patient with Prostate Cancer

Classification	Drug
Antidepressants	Amitriptyline, doxepin
Antihistamines	Chorpheniramine, diphendyramine, hydroxyzine, promethazine
Diabetic agents	Chlorpropamide
Cardiac	Digoxin, dipyridamole
Anihypertensives	Propranolol, clonidine
Sedatives	Barbiturates, chlordiazepoxide, diazepam, flurazepam, meprobamate
Opioids	Meperidine, pentazocine, propoxyphene
Nonsteroidal anti-inflammatory agents	Indomethacin, phenylbutazone
Anticholinergics	Atropine, scopolamine
Antiemetics	Trimethobenzamide, phenothiazine
Antispasmodics	Dicyclomine, hyoscyamine, propantheline, belladonna alkaloids
Antineoplastics	Methotrexate, mitomycin, procarbazine, Ara-C, carmustine, fluorouracil, interferon, interleuken-2, L-asparaginase, prednisone
Corticosteroids	Prednisone, dexamethasone
H² receptor antagonists	Cimetidine
Lithium	
Acetaminophen	
Salicylates	Aspirin
Anticonvulsant agents	Carbamazepine, diphenylhydantoin, phenobarbitone, sodium valproate
Antiparkinson agents	Amantadine, levodopa
Alcohol	

Note. Adapted from Lipowski, Z. (1990). Delirium in geriatric patients. In *Delirium: Acute Confusional States* (pp. 229–276, 413–441). New York: Oxford University Press.

FAMILY/CAREGIVER ISSUES

The term caregiver refers to anyone who provides assistance to someone else who needs it. Informal caregiver is a term used to refer to unpaid individuals such as family members and friends who provide care. The burden of caregiving has been well documented in the literature and results in a greater number of depressive symptoms, anxiety, diminished physical health, financial problems, and disruption in work for the caregiver (Ferrell et al., 1999). The amount of instrumental care needs of the patient strongly relates to family and caregiver psychological distress and burden of care. Patients with prostate cancer who are dying, require varying levels of assistance. The confused or agitated patient places a further strain on the caregiver. Ideally, support of the caregiver should include provisions for adequate homecare, psychological support and bereavement follow-up (Kissane et al., 1998; Smeenk et al., 1998).

HOSPICE CARE

Hospice care is a philosophy of care that can occur in a variety of settings, including the home, hospital or an inpatient hospice unit. Hospice care in the U.S. developed as a grass roots effort to assist terminally-ill patients to die at home. The focus of hospice care is the relief of pain and suffering at the end of life. The patient and family are considered the unit of care, and physical, emotional, social, and spiritual needs are addressed by an interdisciplinary team, including, but not exclusive of, medicine, nursing, social work, and chaplaincy. Bereavement follow-up is an essential component of care as well. Although there are a few inpatient facilities across the U.S., and some hospitals and nursing homes may have hospice beds, the majority of hospice care is delivered in the home.

CONCLUSION

Caring for the patient with prostate cancer at the end of life is a challenge to clinicians today. These patients can be highly symptomatic. Awareness of patterns and sites of metastasis, as well as knowledge of symptom management, will enable clinicians to provide appropriate interventions that may improve quality of life. Caregivers also need support and may need respite care. Skillful and expert palliative care should be the standard of care in this population.

References

Aaronson, N. K. (1988). Quality of life: What is it? How should it be measured? *Oncology, 2*(5), 69–76.

Aaronson, N. K., Ahmedzai, S., Bergman, Bullinger, M., Cull, A., Duez, N. J., Filiberti, A., Fletchtner, H., Fleishman, S. B., de Haes, J. C. J. M., Kassa, S., Klee, M., Osaba, D., Razavi, D., Rofe, P. B., Schraub, S., Sneeuw, K., Sullivan, M., & Takeda F. (1993). The European Organization for the Research of Treatment for Cancer QLQ-C30: A quality of life instrument for use in international clinical trials in oncology. *Journal of the National Cancer Institute, 85,* 365.

Abbou, C. C., Salomon, L., Hoznek, A., Antiphon, P., Cicco, A., Saint, F., Alame, W., Bellot, J., & Chopin, D. K. (2000). Laparoscopic radical prostatectomy: Preliminary results. *Urology, 55*(5), 630–634.

Abel, L. J., Blatt, H. J., Stipetich, R. L., Fuscardo, J. A., Zeroski, D., Miller, S. E., Dorsey, A. T., Butler, W. M., & Merrick, G. S. (1999). Nursing management of patients receiving brachytherapy for early stage prostate cancer. *Clinical Journal of Oncology Nursing, 3*(1), 7–15.

Adami, S. (1997). Bisphosphonates in Prostate carcinoma. *Cancer, 80*(Suppl. 8), 1674–1679.

Adams, M. (1991). Information and education across the phases of cancer care. *Seminars in Oncology Nursing, 7*(2), 105–111.

Adamson, G. M. (1996). The incontinence connection. *Contemporary Long-Term Care, 78,* 129.

Aistars, J. (1987). Fatigue in the cancer patient: A conceptual approach to a clinical problem. *Oncology Nursing Forum, 14*(6), 25–30.

Albertsen, P. C., Fryback, D. G., Storer, B. E., Kolon, T. F., & Fine, J. (1995). Long-term survival among men with conservatively treated localized prostate cancer. *Journal of the American Medical Association, 274*(8), 626–631.

Adelman, R. D., Greene, M. G., & Charon, R. (1987). The physician-elderly patient companion triad in the medical encounter: The development of a conceptual framework and research agenda. *The Gerontologist, 27,* 729–734.

Agency for Health Care Policy and Research (1995). Patient outcomes research team. *Prostate disease.* AHCPR Pub. No. 95-N010. U. S. Department of Health and Human Services. Public Health Service, Agency for Health Care Policy and Research.

Albanes, D., & Taylor, P. R. (1990). International differences in body height and weight and their relationship to cancer incidence. *Nutrition and Cancer, 14,* 69–77.

Albertsen, P. (1996). Screening for prostate cancer is neither appropriate nor cost-effective. *Urology Clinics of North America, 23*(4), 521–530.

Albertsen, P., Aaronson, N., Muller, M., Keller, S., & Ware, J. E. Jr. (1997). Health-related quality of life among patients with metastatic prostate cancer. *Urology, 49*(2), 207–216; discussion: 216–217.

Albertsen, P., Hanley, J., Gleason, D., & Barry, M. J. (1998). Competing risk analysis of men aged 55 to 74 years at diagnosis managed conservatively for clinically localized prostate cancer. *Journal of the American Medical Association, 280*(11), 975–980.

Alliance of Cancer Pain Initiatives Resource Center. Madison, WI. website:aacpi. org.

American Alliance of Cancer Pain Initiatives Resource Center. Madison, WI. website:http://www.aacpi.org.

American Cancer Society (2000). *Cancer facts and figures—2000.* Atlanta, GA: American Cancer Society.

American Cancer Society. (2001). *Cancer facts and figures.* Atlanta, GA: American Cancer Society.

American Cancer Society. *Prostate Cancer Resource Center.* American Cancer Society; 2000. Available www3. cancer. org/cancerinfo/load_cont. asp?

American Geriatric Society Panel on Chronic Pain in Older Persons. (1998). The management of chronic pain in older persons. *JAGS, 46,* 635–651.

American Pain Society (1999). *Principles of analgesic use in the treatment of acute pain and cancer pain.* Glenview, IL.

American Urological Association. (2000). Prostate-Specific Antigen (PSA) best practice policy. *Oncology (Huntington), 14*(2), 267–286.

Andersson, S. O., Wolk, A., Bergstrom, R., Adami, H. O., Engholm, G., Englund, A., & Nyren, O. (1997). Body size and prostate cancer: A 20-year follow-up study among 135,006 Swedish construction workers. *Journal of the American Cancer Institute, 89*(5), 385–389.

Annon, J. S. (1974). *Behavioral treatment of sexual problems* (1st ed.). Hagerstown, MD: Harper & Row.

Annon, J. (1976). The PLISSIT model. A proposed conceptual scheme for behavioral treatment of sexual problems. *Journal of Sex Education & Therapy.*

Arcangeli, G., Giovinazzo, G., Saracino, B., D'Angelo, L., Giannarelli, D., & Micheli, A. (1998). Radiation therapy in the management of symptomatic bone metastases: The effect of total dose and histology on pain relief and response duration. *Int J Radiat Oncol Biol Phys 42*(5), 1119–1126.

Aronson, W. J., & Freeland, S. J. (2000). Editorial: Can we lower the mortality rate of black men with prostate cancer? *The Journal of Urology, 163,* 150–151.

Arterbery, V. E., Frazie, A., Dalmia, P., Siefer, J., Lutz, M., Porter, A. (1997). Quality of life after permanent prostate implant. *Seminars in Surgical Oncology, 1,* 461–464.

Barrett, D. M., & Licht, M. R. (1998). Implantation of the artificial genitourinary sphincter in men and women. In P. C. Walsh, A. B. Retik, E. D. Jr. Vaughan, & A. J. Wein (Eds.), *Campbells' Urology* (7th ed., pp. 1121–1134). Philadelphia, PA: Saunders.

Bates, T. S., Wright, M. P. J., & Gillatt, D. A. (1998). Prevalence and impact of incontinence and impotence following total prostatectomy assessed anonymously by the ICS-Male questionnaire. *European Oncology, 33,* 165–169.

Baum, N., Appell, R. A., & Moss, H (1994). Helping incontinent patients resume activity. *Physician Sportsmedicine 22,* 70.

Bazinet, M., Meshref, A. W., Trudel, C., Aronson, S., Peloguin, F., Nachabe, M., Begin, L. R., & Elhilali, M. M. (1994). Prospective evaluation of prostate-specific antigen density and systematic biopsies for early detection of prostatic carcinoma. *Urology, 43,* 44–51.

Beahrs, O. H., Henson, D. E., Hutter, P. V. P., & Kennedy, B. J. (1992). *Manual for staging of cancer* (4th ed., pp. 181–186). Philadelphia: J. B. Lippincott.

Beck, J. R., Kattan, M. W., & Miles, B. J. (1994). A critique of the decision analysis for clinically localized prostate cancer. *The Journal of Urology, 152,* 1894–1904.

Becker, M. H. (1974). *The health belief model and personal health behavior.* Thorofare, NJ: Charles B. Slack.

Beisecker, A. E. (1988). Aging and desire for information and input in medical decisions: Patient consumerism in medical encounters. *The Gerontologist, 28,* 330–335.

Benoit, R. M., Naslund, M. J., & Cohen, J. K. (2000). Complications after prostate brachytherapy in the Medicare population. *Urology, 55*(1), 91–96.

Benson, M. C., Whang, I. S., Olsson, C. A., McMahon, D. J., & Cooner, W. H. (1992). The use of Prostate-specific antigen density to prostate-specific antigen. *Journal of Urology, 147,* 817–821.

Berenson, J. R., Lichtenstein, A., Porter, L., Dimopoulos, M., Bordoni,

R., George, S., Lipton, A., Keller, A., Ballester, O., Kovacs, M. J., Blacklock, H. A., Bell, R., Simeone, J., Reitsma, D. J., Heffernan, M., & Seaman, J. (1996). Efficacy of pamidronate in reducing skeletal events in patients with advanced multple myeloma. *New Eng J Med, 334*(8), 488–493.

Billhorn, D. R. (1994). Sexuality and the chronically ill older adult, *Geriatric Nursing 15,* 106–108.

Bishop, D. T., & Skolnick, M. H. (1984). Genetic epidemiology of cancer in Utah genealogies: A prelude to the molecular genetics of common cancers. *Journal of Cellular Physiology, 3*(suppl), 63–77.

Blair, A., & Zahn, S. H. (1991). Cancer among farmers. *Occupational Medicine, 6,* 335–354.

Blanchard, C. G., Labreque, M. S., Ruckdeschel, J. C., & Blanchard, E. B. (1988). Information and decision making preferences in hospitalized adult cancer patients. *Social Science & Medicine, 27,* 1139–1145.

Blasko, J. C., Grimm, P. D., Ragde, H., & Schumacher, D. (1997). Implant therapy for localized prostate cancer. In M. S. Ernstoff, J. A. Heaney, & R. E. Peschel (Eds.), *Urologic cancer.* Cambridge: Blackwell Science.

Blasko, J. C., Ragde, H., Grimm, P. D., Cavanagh, W., & Kenny, G. (1995). Transperineal palladium-103 brachytherapy for prostate cancer. *Journal of Urology, 153,* 6–26.

Blasko, J. C., & Wallner, K. (1997). Brachytherapy for early prostate cancer—Part II: Clinical experience and future directions. *Proceedings of the 39th Annual Meeting American Society for Therapeutic Radiology and Oncology* (pp. 1–13). Orlando, FL.

Blasko, J. C., Ragde, H., & Grimm, P. D. (1991). Transperineal ultrasound-guided implantation of the prostate: morbidity and complications. *Scandinavian Journal of Urology & Nephrology, 137*(Suppl), 113–118.

Blasko, J. C., Wallner, K. E., Grimm, P. D., & Ragde, H. (1995). PSA-based disease control following ultrasound guided I-125 implantation for T1/T2 prostatic carcinoma. *Journal of Urology, 154,* 1096–1099.

Block, S. D. (2000). Assessing and managing depression in the terminally ill patient. ACP-ASIM End-of-Life Care Consensus Panel. American College of Physicians—American Society of Internal Medicine. *Annals of Internal Medicine, 132,* 209–218.

Boccardo, F. (2000). Hormone therapy of prostate cancer: Is there a role for antiandrogen monotherapy? *Critical Revue Oncology Hematology, 35*(2), 121–132.

Bookbinder, M., Coyle, N., Kiss, M., Layman Goldstein, M., Holritz, K., Thaler, H., Gianella, A., Derby, S., Brown, M., Racolin, A., Ho, M. N., & Portenoy, R. K. (1996). Implementing national standards

for cancer pain management: Program model and evaluation. *J Pain Symptom Manage, 12,* 334–347.
Borboroglu, P. G., Sands, J. P., Roberts, J. L., & Amling, C. L. (2000). Risk factors for vesicourethral anastomic structure after radical prostatectomy. *Urology, 56,* 96–100.
Bordinazzo, R., Benecchi, L., Bookbinder, M., Coyle, N., Kiss, M., Layman, G. M., Holritz, K., Thaler, H., Gianella, A., Derby, S., Brown, M., Racolin, A., Ho, M. N., & Portenoy, R. K. (1996). Implementing National Standards for Cancer Pain Management: Program Model and Evaluation. *J Pain Symptom Manage, 12,* 334–347.
Borghede, G., Karlsson, J., & Sullivan, M. (1997). Quality of life in patients with prostatic cancer: Results from a Swedish population study. *Journal of Urology, 158,* 1477–1486.
Borre M., Nerstrom, B., & Overgaard, J. (2000). Association between immunohistochemical expression of vascular endothelial growth factor (VEGF), VEGF-expressing neuroendocrine-differentiated tumor cells, and outcome in prostate cancer patients subjected to watchful waiting. *Clinical Cancer Research, 6,* 1882–1890.
Borre, M., Offersen, B. V., Nerstrom, B., & Overgaard, J. (1998). Microvessel density predicts survival in prostate cancer patients subjected to watchful waiting. *British Journal of Cancer, 78,* 940–944.
Bostwick, D. G., MacLennan, G. T., & Larson, T. R. (1999). American Cancer Society. *Prostate cancer: What every man and his family needs to know* (rev. ed.). New York: Villard.
Brawer, M. K. (1999). Prostate-specific antigen: Current status. *CA Cancer Journal for Clinicians, 49,* 264–281.
Brawer, M. K., Arambura, E. A., Chen, G. L., Preston, S. D., & Ellis, W. J. (1993). The inability of prostate specific antigen index to enhance the predictive the value of prostate specific antigen in the diagnosis of prostatic carcinoma. *Journal of Urology, 150,* 369–373.
Brawer, M. K., Catalona, W., & McConnell, J. (1992). Prostate cancer: Is screening the answer? *Patient Care, 26*(16), 55–68.
Brawley, O. W., & Thompson, I. M. (1994). Chemoprevention of prostate cancer. *Urology, 43*(5), 594–597.
Brawley, O. W., Knopf, K., & Thompson, I. (1998). The epidemiology of prostate cancer, Part II: The risk factors. *Seminars in Urologic Oncology, 16*(4), 193–201.
Brawley, O. W., Knopf, K., & Thompson, I. (1999). The epidemiology of prostate cancer. Part II—The risk factors. *Seminars in Urologic Oncology 16,* 193–201.
Breitbart, W., Rosenfeld, B., Roth, A., Smith, M. J., Cohen, K., & Passik, S. (1997). The Memorial Delirium Assessment Scale. *J Pain Symptom Manage, 13,* 128–137.

Breitbart, W., & Jacobsen, P. B. (1996). Psychiatric symptom management in terminal care. *Clin Geriatr Med, 12,* 329–347.

Breitbart, W., Breura, E., Chochinov, H., & Lynch. M. (1995). Neuropsychiatric syndromes and psychological symptoms in patients with advanced cancer. *J Pain Symptom Manage, 10,* 131–141.

Breslow, R. A., & Weed, D. L. (1998). Review of epidemiologic studies of alcohol and prostate cancer: 1971–1996. *Nutrition and Cancer, 30,* 1–13.

Brown, T., & Griffiths, P. (1986). Cancer self help groups: An inside view. *British Medical Journal, 292,* 1503–1504.

Brudage, M. D., Crook, J. M., & Lukka. H. (1998). Use of Strontium-89 in endocrine-refractory prostate cancer metastatic to bone. Provincial Genitourinary Cancer Disease Site Group. *Cancer Prev Control 2*(2), 79–87.

Bruera, E., & MacDonald, R. N. (1988). Asthenia in patients with advanced cancer. *J Pain Symptom Manage, 3,* 9–14.

Burklow, J. (1992). Doctors concerned about age bias in cancer treatment. *Journal of the National Cancer Institute, 84,* 391.

CA: A Cancer Journal for Clinicians. (2000). *Cancer Statistics, 50*(1).

Carlsson, A. M. (1983). Assessment of chronic pain. I. Aspects of the reliability and validity of the visual analogue scale. *Pain, 16*(1), 87–101.

Carroll-Johnson, R. M., Mahon, S. M., & Jennings-Dozier, K. M. (Eds.). (2000). Cancer prevention and early detection: Oncology nursing's next frontier. *Oncology Nursing Forum, 27*(Suppl. 9), 1–63.

Carson, C. C., Mulcahy, J. J., Govier, F. E. (2000). Efficacy, safety and patient satisfaction outcomes of the AMS 700CX inflatable penile prosthesis: Results of a long term multicenter study. AMS 700 CX Study Group. *Journal of Urology, 164*(2) 376–380.

Carter, B. J. (1997). Women's experiences of lymphedema. *Oncol Nurs Forum, 24,* 875–882.

Carter, H. B., & Partin, A. W. (1998). Diagnosis and staging of prostate cancer. In P. C. Walsh, A. B. Retik, E. D. Jr. Vaughan, & A. J. Wein, *Campbell's Urology* (7th ed., pp. 2519–2537).

Carter, B. S., Beaty, T. H., Steinberg, G. D., Childs, B., & Walsh, P. C. (1992). Mendelian inheritance of familial prostate cancer. *Proceedings of the National Academy of Science, USA, 89,* 3367–3371.

Carter, B. S., Beaty, T. H., Steinberg, G. D., Childs, B., & Walsh, P. C. (1992). Mendelian inheritance of familial prostate cancer. *Proceedings of the National Academy of Science, USA, 89,* 3367–3371.

Carter, H. B., & Partin, A. W. (1998). Diagnosis and staging of prostate cancer. In P. C. Walsh, A. B. Retik, E. D. Jr. Vaughan, & A. J. Wein, *Campbell's urology* (7th ed., pp. 2519–2537). Philadelphia: Saunders.

Carter, H. B., Pearson, J. D., Metter, E. J., Brant, L. J., Chen, D. W.,

Andres, R., Fozard, J. D., & Walsh, P. C. (1992). Longitudinal evaluation of prostate-specific antigen levels in men with and without prostatic disease. *Journal of the American Medical Association, 272*, 813–814.

Cash, J. C., & Dattoli, M. J. (1997). Management of patients receiving transperineal palladium-103 prostate implants. *Oncology Nursing Forum, 24*(8), 1361–1367.

Cassileth, B. R., Soloway, M. S., Vogelzang, N. J., Schellhammer, P. S., Seidmon, E. J., Hait, H., & Kennealey, G. T. (1989). Patients' choice of treatment in stage D prostate cacner. *Urology, 33*(5 supplement), 57–62.

Cassileth, B. R. Zupkis, R. V., Sutton-Smith, K., March, V. (1980). Information participation preferences among cancer patients. *Annals of Internal Medicine, 92*, 832–836.

Catalona, W. J., Ramos, C. G., & Carvahal, G. F. (1999). Contemporary results of anatomic radical prostatectomy. *Cancer: A Cancer Journal for Clinicians, 49*(5), 282–296.

Catalona, W. J., Richie, J. P., Ahmann, F. R., Hudson, M. A., Scardino, P. T., Flanigan, R. C., dekernion, J. B., Ratliff, T. L., Kavoussi, L. R., & Dalkin, B. L. (1994). Comparison of digital rectal examination and serum prostate specific antigen in the early detection of prostate cancer: Results of a multicenter clinical trial of 6,630 men. *Journal of Urology, 151*, 1283–1290.

Catalona, W. J., Smith, D. S., Wolfert, R. L., Wang, T. J., Rittenhouse, H. G., Ratliff, T. L., & Nadler, R. B. (1995). Evaluation of percentage of free serum prostatic-specific antigen to improve specificity of prostate cancer screening. *Journal of the American Medical Association, 274*, 1214–1220.

Catalona, W. J., Caravalhal, G. F., Mager, D. E., & Smith, D. S. (1999). Potenecy, continence and complication rates in 1,870 consecutive retropubic prostatectomies. *Journal of Urology, 162*, 433–438.

Cazzaniga, A., Vercesi, A., & Privitera, O. (1994). Ureteral obstruction associated with prostate cancer: The outcome after ultrasonographic percutaneous nephrostomy. *Arch Ital Urol Androl, 66*(suppl), 101–106.

Cella, D., Tulsky, D., Gray, G., Sarafian, B., Linn, E., Bonomi, A., Silberman, M., Yellen, S., Winicour, P., Brannon. J, et al (1993). The Functional Assessment of Cancer Therapy scale: Development and validation of the general measure. *Journal of Clinical Oncology, 11*(3), 570–579.

Cespedes, R. D., Leng, W. W., & McGuire, E. J. (1999). Collagen injection therapy for postprostatectomy incontinence. *Urology, 54*, 597–602.

Cha, C. M., Potters, L., Ashley, R., Freemman, K., Wang, X. H., Waldbaum,

R., & Leibel, S. (1999). Isotope selection for patients undergoing prostate brachytherapy. *International Journal of Radiation Oncology, Biology & Physics, 45*(2), 391–395.

Chan, J. M., Stampfer, M. J., & Giovannucci, E. L. (1998). What causes prostate cancer? A brief summary of the epidemiology. *Seminars in Cancer Biology, 8,* 263–273.

Chiou, R. K., Chang, W. Y., & Horn, J. J. (1990). Ureteral obstruction associated with prostate cancer: The outcome after percutaneous nephrostomy. *J Urol, 143,* 957–959.

Chochinov, H. M., Wilson, K. G., Enns, M., & Lander, S. (1994). Prevalence of depression in the terminally ill: Effects of diagnostic criteria and symptom threshold judgements. *Am. J of Psychiatry, 151,* 537–540.

Chochinov, H. M., Wilson, K. G., Enns, M., & Lander, S. (1997). "Are you depressed?" Screening for depression in the terminally ill. *Am. J of Psychiatry, 154,* 674–676.

Chodak, G. W., Thisted, R. A., Gerber, G. S., Johansson, J. E., Adolfsson, J., Jones, G. W., Chisholm, G. D., Moskovitz, B., Livne, P. M., & Warner, J. (1994). Results of conservative management of clinically localized prostate cancer. *N Engl J Med, 330,* 242–248.

Ciaramella, A., & Poli, P. (2001). Assessment of depression among cancer patients: The role of pain, cancer type and treatment. *Psychooncology, 10,* 156–165.

Clark, J., Wray, N., & Ashton, C. (2001). Living with treatment decisions: Regrets and quality of life among men treated for metastatic prostate cancer. *Journal of Clinical Oncology, 19*(1), 72–80.

Clark, L. C., Dalkin, B., Krongrad, A., Combs, G. F., Jr., Turnbull, B. W., Slate, E. H., Witherington, R., Herlong, J. H., Janoska, E., Carpenter, D., Borosso, C., Falk, S., & Rounder, J. (1998). Decreased incidence of prostate cancer with selenium supplementation: Results of a double-blind cancer prevention trial. *British Journal of Urology, 81*(5), 730–734.

Clarke, N. W., McCLure, J., & George, N. J. R. (1992). Clinical and metabolic effects of disodium pamidronate in metastatic prostate cancer. In O. L. M. Biijvoet & A. Lipton (Eds.), *Osteoclastic inhibition in the management of malignancy-related bone disorders* (pp. 54–63). Toronto: Hogrefe and Huber.

Clark, P. M., & Lacasse, C. (1998). Cancer-related fatigue: Clinical practice issues. *Clinical Journal of Oncology Nursing, 2*(2), 45–53.

Cleeland, C. S., Gonin, R., Hatfield, A. K., Edmonson, J. H., Blum, R. H., Stewart, J. A., & Padya, K. J. (1994). Pain and its treatment inoutpatients with metastatic cancer. *N Engl J Med, 330*(9), 592–596.

Chao, C. K. S., Perez, C. A., & Brady, L. W. (1999). Prostate. *Radiation oncology: Management decisions.* Philadelphia: Lippincott.

Coe, R. M., & Prendergast, C. (1985). Research note. The formation of coalitions: Interactions in triads. *Sociology of Health & Medicine, 7,* 236–247.

Cohen, J. H., Kristal, A. R., & Stanford, J. L. (2000). Fruit and vegetable intakes and prostate cancer risk. *Journal of the National Cancer Institute, 92*(1), 61–68.

Coley, C. M., Barry, M. J., & Mulley, A. G. (1997). Screening for prostate cancer. *Annals of Internal of Medication, 126,* 480–484.

Coley, C. M., Barry, M. J., Fleming, C., Fahs, M., & Mulley, A. G. (1997). Early detection of prostate cancer: II Estimating the risks, benefits, and cost. *Annals of Internal Medicine, 126,* 468–479.

Coley, C. M., Barry, M. J., Fleming, C., & Mulley, A. G. (1997). Early detection of prostate cancer part I: Prior probability and effectiveness of tests. *Annals of Internal Medicine, 126,* 394–406.

Coley, C. M., Barry, M. J., Fleming, C., Fahs, M., & Mulley, A. G. (1997b). Early detection of prostate cancer: Part II: Estimating the risks, benefits and costs. *Annals of Internal Medicine, 126*(6), 468–479.

Collins, M. M., Roberts, R. G., Oesterling, J. E., Wasson, J. H., & Barry, M. J. (1998). Prostate cancer screening and beliefs about treatment efficacy: A national survey of primary care physicians and urologists. *American Journal of Medicine, 104,* 526–532.

Colombel, M, Mallame W & Abbou, CC. (1997). Influence of urological complications on the prognosis of prostate cancer. *Eur Urol, 13*(suppl 3), 21–24.

Cooney, K. A., McCarthy, J. D., Lange, E., Huang, L., Meisfeldt, S., Montie, J. E., Oesterling, J. E., Sandler, H. M., & Lange, K. (1997). Prostate cancer susceptibility locus on chromosome 1q: A confirmatory study. *Journal of the National Cancer Institute, 89,* 955–959.

Coreil, J., & Behal, R. (1999). Man to man prostate cancer support groups. *Cancer Practice, 7*(3), 122–129.

Counter, S. F., Froese, D. P., & Hart, M. J. (1999). Prospective evaluation of formalin therapy for radiation proctitis. *The American Journal of Surgery, 177*(5), 396–398.

Coyle N, Adelhardt J, Foley K & Portenoy R. (1990). Character of terminal illness in the advanced cancer patient: Pain and other symptoms during the last four weeks of life. *J Pain and Sympt Manage, (5)*2, 83–93.

Crawford, E. D. et al. (1989). A controlled trial of leuprolide with and without flutamide in prostatic carcinoma. *New England Journal of Medicine, 321,* 419.

Crawford, E. D., Eisenberger, M., McLeod, D. G., Wilding, G., & Blumenstein, B. A. (1997). Comparison of bilateral orchiectomy with or without flutamide for the treatment of patients with stage

D2 adenocarcinoma of the prostate: Results of the NCI Intergroup Study 0105. *British Journal of Urology, 80,* 1092A.

Crosson, K. (1984). Cancer patient education: What, where and by whom? *Health Education Quarterly, 10*(suppl), 19–29.

Cryer, B., & Feldman, M. (1998). Cyclooxygenase-1 and Cyclooxygenase-2 selectivity of widely used Nonsteroidal Anti-Inflammatory drugs. *Am J Med, 104,* 413–421.

Davis, W., Kuban, D. A., Lynch, D. F., & Schellhammer, P. F. (2000). Quality of life after radical prostatectomy vs. brachytherapy for localized prostate cancer. *The Journal of Urology, 163*(suppl. 4), abstract #286.

Davidson, P. J. T., van den Ouden, D., & Schroeder, F. H. (1996). Radical prostatectomy: Prospective assessment of mortality and morbidity. *European Oncology, 29,* 168–173.

Davis, D. L. (1998). Prostate cancer treatment with radioactive seed implantation. *AORN Journal, 68*(1), 18–40.

Davison, B. J., Degner, L. F., & Morgan, T. R. (1995). Information on decision-making preferences of men with prostate cancer. *Oncology Nursing Forum, 22,* 1401–1408.

Davison, B. J., & Degner, L. F. (1997). Empowerment of men newly diagnosed with prostate cancer. *Cancer Nursing, 20,* 187–196.

Daw, H. A., & Peereboom, D. M. (2000). Prostate cancer: Endocrine therapy. In E. D. Kursh & J. C. Ulchaker (Eds.), *Office Urology* (pp. 291–301). Totowa, NJ: Humana Press.

Dean, G. E., & Anderson, P. R. (2001). Fatigue. In B. R. Ferrell & N. Coyle (Eds.), *Textbook of palliative nursing* (pp. 91–100). New York: Oxford University Press.

Dearnaley, D. P., Khoo, V. S., Norman, A. R., Meyer, L., Nahum, A., Tait, D, Yarnold,J., & Horwich, A. (1999). Comparison of radiation side-effects of conformal and conventional radiotherapy in prostate cancer: A randomised trial. *The Lancet, 353*(9149), 267–272.

Degner, L. F., & Russel, C. A. (1988). Preferences of treatment control among adults with cancer. *Research in Nursing & in Health, 11,* 367–374.

Degner, L. F., & Sloan, J. A. (1992). Decision making during serious illness: What role do patients really want to play? *Journal of Clinical Epidemiology, 45,* 941–950.

Delfino, R. J., Ferrini, R. L., Taylor, T. H., Howe, S., & Anton-Culver, H. (1998). Demographic differences in prostate cancer incidence and stage: An examination of population diversity. *American Journal of Preventive Medicine, 114,* 96–102.

DeMarco, R. T., Bihrle, R., & Foster, R. S. (2000). Early catheter removal following radical retropubic prostatectomy. *Seminars in Urologic Oncology, 18*(1) 57–59.

Dennis, L. K. (2000). Meta-analysis for combining relative risks of alcohol consumption and prostate cancer. *Prostate, 42*(1), 56–66.

Derby, S. E. (1991). Ageism in cancer care of the elderly. *Oncology Nursing Forum, 18,* 921–926.

Derby S, & Portenoy R. (1997). Assessment and management of opioid-induced constipation. In R. K. Portenoy & E. Bruera (Eds.), *Topics in Palliative Care* (vol. 1, pp. 95–112). New York: Oxford University Press.

Dodd, M. J. (1984). Patterns of self-care in cancer patients receiving radiation therapy. *Oncology Nursing Forum, 10,* 23–27.

Doherty, K., & Breslin, S. (1996). Prostate cancer: An update on screening and management. In S. M. Hubbard, M. Goodman, & M. T. Knobf (Eds.), *Oncology nursing updates: Patient treatment and support,* (pp. 1–13). Philadelphia: Lippincott-Raven.

Dole, E. J., & Holdsworth, M. T. (1997). Nilutamide: An antiandrogen for the treatment of prostate cancer. *The Annals of Pharmacotherapy,* January (31), 65–75.

Donahue, M. P. (1985). *Nursing the finest art: An illustrated history.* St. Louis, MO: The C. V. Mosby Company.

Drench, M. E., & Losee, R. H. (1996). Sexuality and sexual capacities of elderly people. *Rehabilitation Nursing, 2,* 118–123.

Dvoracek, J. (1998). Adenocarcinoma of the prostate. *Casopis Lekaru Ceskych, 137,* 515–521.

Earnest, D. L. (1991). Radiation proctitis. *Practical Gastroenterology, 15*(1), 15–21.

Egbert, A. M. (1996). Postoperative pain management in the frail elderly. *Clin Ger Med, 12*(3), 582–600.

Ekman, P. (1999). Genetic and environmental factors in prostate cancer genesis: Identifying high-risk cohorts. *European Urology, 35,* 362–369.

Endicott, J. (1984). Measurement of depression in patients with cancer. *Cancer, 53*(suppl), 2243–2248.

Epstein, B. E., & Hanks, G. E. (1992). Prostate cancer: Evaluation and radiotherapeutic management. *CA: A Cancer Journal for Clinicians, 42*(4), 223–240.

Ernst, D. S. (1998). Role of bisphosphonates and other bone resorption inhibitorls in metastatic bone pain. In R. K. Portenoy & E Bruera (Eds.). *Topics in palliative care* (vol 3). New York: Oxford University Press.

Eschenbach. (1999). Prostate cancer. *CA: A Cancer Journal for Clinicians, 49.*

Esper, P., Hampton, J. N., Smith, D. C., & Pienta, K. J. (1999). Quality-of-life evaluation in patients receiving treatment for advanced prostate cancer. *Oncology Nursing Forum. 26*(1), 107–112.

Esper, P. & Redman, B. G. (1999). Supportive care, pain management and quality of life in advanced prostate cancer. *Urol Clin of N America, 26*(2), 375–389.

Fainsinger, R., Miller, M. J., Bruera, E., & Hanson, J., & McEachern, T. (1991). Symptom control during the last week of life on a palliative care unit. *J Palliat Care, 7*(1), 5–11

Fair, W. R., Fleshner, N. E., & Heston, W. (1997). Cancer of the prostate: A nutritional disease? *Urology, 50,* 840–848.

Fawzy, F. I., Fawzy, N. W., Hyun, C. S., Elashoff, R.. Guthrie, D., Fahey, J. L., & Morton, D. L. (1993). Malignant melanoma. Effects of an early structured psychiatric intervention, coping, and affective state on recurrence and survival 6 years later. *Archives of General Psychiatry, 50*(9), 681–689.

Fayers, P., & Jones, D. (1983). Measuring and analysing quality of life in cancer clinical trials: A review. *Statistics in Medicine, 2,* 429–446.

Feldman-Stewart, D., Brubdage, M. D., Hayter, C., Nickel, J. C., Downes, H., Mackillop, W. J. (2000). What questions do patients with curable prostate cancer want answered? *Medical Decision Making, 20,* 7–19.

Feneley, M. R, Gillatt, D. A., Hehir, M., & Kirby, R. S. (1996). A review of radical prostatectomy from three centers in the UK Clinical presentation and outcome. *British Journal of Urology, 78,* 911–920.

Feng, M. I., Huang, S., Kaptein, J., Kaswick, J., & Aboseif, S. (2000). Effect of sildenafil citrate on post-radical prostatectomy erectile dysfunction. *Journal of Urology, 164,* (6), 1935–1938.

Ferrans, C. E. (1990). Quality of life: Conceptual issues. *Seminars in Oncology Nursing, 6,* 248–254.

Ferrans, C. E. (1996). Development of a conceptual model of quality of life. *Scholarly Inquiry for Nursing Practice, 10,* 293–304.

Ferrans, C. E., & Powers, M. J. (1985). Quality of life index: Development and psychometric properties. *ANS, 8,* 15–21.

Ferrell, B. R., Grant, M., Borneman, T., Juarez, G., & Ter Veer, A. (1999). Family caregiving in cancer pain management. *J of Palliative Med, 2,* 185–195.

Ferrell, B. R., Grant, M., Richey, K. J., Ropchan, R., & Rivera, L. M. (1993). The pain resource nurse training program: A unique approach to pain management. *J Pain Symptom Manage, 8,* 549–556.

Ferrell, B., Wisdom, C., Wenzl, C., & Brown, J. (1989). Effects of controlled-release morphine on quality of life for cancer pain. *Oncology Nursing Forum, 16,* 521–526.

Ficazzola, M., & Nitti, V. (1998). The etiology of post-radical prostatectomy incontinence and correlation of symptoms with urodynamic findings. *Journal of Urology, 160*(4), 1317–1320.

Fitch, M. I., Gray, R., Franssen, E., & Johnson, B. (2000). Men's perspectives on the impact of prostate cancer: Implications for oncology nurses. *Oncology Nursing Forum* (pp. 1255–1263). Pittsburgh, PA: Oncology Press.

Flanagan, J. (1982). Measurement of quality of life: Current state of the art. *Archives in Physical Medicine & Rehabilitation, 63*(2), 56–59.

Fleming, C., Wasson, J. H. Albertsen, P. C., Barry, M. J., & Wennberg, J. E. (1993). A decision analysis of alternative treatment strategies for clinically localized prostate cancer. Prostate Patient Outcomes Research Team. *Journal of the American Medical Association, 269*, 2650–2658.

Foreman M. D. (1993). Acute confusion in the elderly. *Annual Rev of Nurs Research, 11*, 3–30.

Fowler, F. J. (1995). Prostate conditions, treatment decisions, and patient preferences (editorial). *Journal of the American Geriatrics Society, 43*, 1058–1060.

Fowler, F. J. Jr, Barry, M., Lu-Yao, G., Roman, A., Wasson, J., & Wennberg, J. (1993). Patient-reported complications and follow-up treatment after radical prostatectomy. The National Medicare Experience: 1988–1990 (updated June 1993). *Urology, 42*(6), 622–629.

Fowler, F. J., Barry, M. J., Lu-Yao, G., Wasson, J., & Bin, L. (1996). Outcomes of external beam radiation therapy for prostate cancer: A study of Medicare beneficiaries in three surveillance, epidemiology, and end results areas. *Journal of Clinical Oncology, 14*, 2258–2265.

Fowler, J. E., Jr., & Bigler, S. A. (1999). A prospective study of the serum prostate specific antigen concentrations and Gleason histologic scores of black and white men with prostate carcinoma. *Cancer, 86*, 836–841.

Fowler, F. J Jr., Bin, L., Collins, M. M., Roberts, R. G., Oesterling, J. E., Wasson, J. H., & Barry, M. J. (1998). Prostate cancer screening and beliefs about treatment efficacy: A national survey of primary care physicians and urologists. *American Journal of Medicine, 104*, 526–532.

Fowler, F. J., McNaughton, Collins, M., Albertsen, P. C., Zietman, A., Elliott, D. B., & Barry, M. J. (2000). Comparison of recommendations by urologists and radiation oncologists for treatment of clinically localized prostate cancer. *Journal of the American Medical Association, 283*, 3217–3222.

Frank, I., Graham, S., & Nabors, W. (1991). Urologic and male genital cancers. In A. Holleb, D. Fink, & G. Murphy (Eds.), *American Cancer Society textbook of clinical oncology* (pp. 271–289). Atlanta, GA. American Cancer Society.

Frank-Stromborg, M., & Cohen, R. (1991). Evaluating written patient education materials. *Seminars in Oncology Nursing, 7*(2), 125–134.

Freeman, H. P. (1989). Cancer and the socioeconomically disadvantaged. *Cancer Journal for Clinicians, 39*(5), 263–295.

Frydenberg, M., Stricker, P. D., & Kaye, K. W. (1997). Prostate cancer diagnosis and management. *Lancet, 349*, 1681–1687.

Fulfaro, F., Casuccio, C., Ticozzi, C. & Ripamonti, C. (1998). The role of bisphosphonates in the treatment of painful metastatic bone disease: A review of phase III trial. *Pain, 78*, 157–169.

Galasko, C. S. B. (1982). Mechanisms of lytic and blastic metastatic disease of bone. *Clin Orthop, 169*, 20–27.

Ganem, J. P., Lucey, D. T., Janosko, E. O., & Carson, C. C. (1998). Unusual complications of the vacuum erection device. *Urology, 51*(4), 627–631.

Gann, P. H., Ma, J., Giovannucci, E., Willet, W., Sacks, F. M., Hennekens, C. H., & Stampfer, M. J. (1999). Lower prostate cancer risk in men with elevated plasma lycopene levels: Results of a prospective analysis. *Cancer Research, 59*(6), 1225–1230.

Ganz, P. A., Schag, C. A. C., Lee, J. J., & Sim, M. S. (1992). The CARES: A generic measure of health-related quality of life for patients with cancer. *Qualitative Life Research, 1,* 19–29.

Gardner, T. A., Bissonett, E. A., Petroni, G. R., McClain, R., Sokoloff, M. H., & Thodorescu, D. (2000). Surgical and postoperative factors affecting length of hospital stay after radical

Garfunkel, L. (1991). Statistics and trends. In A. I. Holleb, D. J. Fink, & G. P. Murphy (Eds.), *Textbook of clinical oncology* (pp. 1–6). Atlanta, GA: American Cancer Society.

Garnick, M. B. (1993). Prostate cancer: Screening, diagnosis, and management. *Annals of Internal Medicine, 118,* 804–818

Garnick, M. (1994). The dilemmas of prostate cancer. *Scientific American, 270,* 72–81.

Gelblum, D. Y., & Potters. L. (2000). Rectal complications associated with transperineal interstitial brachytherapy for prostate cancer. *Internal Journal of Radiation Oncology Biology & Physics, 48*(1), 119–124.

Gelfand, D., Parzuchowski, J., Cort, M., & Powell, I. (1995). Digital rectal examinations and prostate cancer screening: Attitudes of African American men. *Oncology Nursing Forum, 22,* 1253–1255.

Gerard, M. J., & Frank-Stromborg, M. (1998). Screening for prostate cancer in asymptomatic men: Clinical, legal and ethical implications. *Oncology Nursing Forum, 25*(9), 1561–1568.

Gerber, G. S., & Chodak, G. W. (1993). Transrectal prostatis ultrasound and biopsy. In S. Das & E. D. Crawford (Eds.), *Cancer of the prostate* (pp. 101–117). Marcel Decker: NY.

Germino, B. B., Mishel, M. H., Belyea, M., Harris, L., Ware, A., &

Mohler, J. (1998). Uncertainty in prostate cancer. Ethnic and family patterns. *Cancer Practice, 6,* 107–113.

Gibbons, R. P: Radical Perineal Prostatectomy. In P. C.Walsh, A. B. Retik, E. D. Vaughan, A. J. Wein, Jr. (Eds.), *Campbells' Urology* (7th ed., pp. 2589–2604). Philadelphia, PA. Saunders.

Gilliland, F., Hoffman, R., Hamilton, A., Albertsen, P., Eley, J., Harlan, Stanford, J., Hunt, W., Potosky, A., & Stephenson, R. (1999). Predicting extracapsular extension of prostate cancer in men treated with radical prostatectomy: Results from the population based prostate cancer outcomes study. *Journal of Urology, 162*(4), 1341–1345.

Gilson, A. M., & Joranson. D. E. (2001). Controlled substance and pain management: Changes in knowledge and attitudes of medical regulators. *J Pain Sypmtom Manage, 21,* 227–237.

Giovannucci, E., Ascherio, A., Rimm, E. B., Colditz, G. A., Stampfer, M. J., & Willett, W. C. (1993). A prospective cohort study of vasectomy and prostate cancer in U.S. men. *Journal of the American Medical Association, 269,* 873–877.

Giovannucci, E. (1995). Epidemiologic characteristics of prostate cancer. *Cancer, 7*(7), (suppl.), 1766–1777.

Giovannucci, E. (1996). How is individual risk for prostate cancer assessed? *Hematology/Oncology Clinics of North America, 10*(3), 537–548.

Giovannucci, E., Rimm, E. B., Colditz, G. A., Stampfer, M. J., Ascherio, A., Chute, C. C., & Willett, W. C. (1993). A prospective study of dietary fat and risk of prostate cancer. *Journal of the National Cancer Institute, 85,* 1571–1579.

Giovannucci, E., Rimm, E. B., Stampfer, M . J., Colditz, G. A., & Willett. W. C. (1997). Height, body weight, and risk of prostate cancer. *Cancer Epidemiology, Biomarkers and Prevention, 6*(8), 557–563.

Giovannucci, E., Tosteson, T. D., Speizer, F. E., Ascherio, A., Vessey, M. P., & Colditz, G. A. (1993). A retrospective cohort study of vasectomy and prostate cancer in U.S. men. *Journal of the American Medical Association, 269,* 878–882.

Glaus, A., Crow, R., & Hammond, S. (1996). A qualitative study to explore the concept of fatigue/tiredness in cancer patients and in healthy individuals. *Supportive Care in Cancer, 4,* 82–96.

Gleason, D., & Mellinger, G. (1974). Prediction of prognosis for prostatic adenocarcinoma by combined histological grading and clinical staging. *Journal of Urology, 111*(1), 58–64.

Gohagan, J. K., Prorok, P. C., Kramer, B. S., & Cornett, J. E. (1994). Prostate cancer screening in the prostate, lung, colorectal, and ovarian cancer screening trial of the National Cancer Institute. *Journal of Urology, 152,* 1905–1909.

Goodyear, M., & Fraumeni, M. (1996). Incorporating quality of life assessment into clinical cancer trials. In B. Spilker (Ed.), *Quality of life and pharmacoeconomics in clinical trials* (2nd ed). Philadelphia: Lippincott-Raven Publishers.

Gordon, D. B., Dahl, J. L., & Stevenson, K. K. (1996). *Building an institutional commitment of pain management.* Madison, WI: UW Board of Regents.

Gray, R. E., Fitch, M. I., Phillips, C., Labrecque, M., & Klotz, L. (1999). Presurgery experiences of prostate cancer patients and their spouses. *Cancer Practice, 7,* 130–135.

Greene, M. G., Majewrovitz, S. D., Adelman, R. D., & Rizzo, C. (1986). The effects of the presence of a third person on the physician-older patient medical interview. *Journal of the American Geriatrics Society, 42,* 413–419.

Greenlee, R. T., Hill-Harmon, M. B., Murray, T., & Thun, M. (2001). Cancer statistics, 2001. *CA: A Cancer Journal for Clinicians, 51*(1), 15–36.

Greenlee, R. T., Murray, T., Bolden, S., & Wingo, P. A. (2000). Cancer statistics, 2000. *Ca:A Cancer Journal for Clinicians, 50*(1), 7–33.

Gregoire, I., Kalogeropoulos, D., & Corcos, J. (1997). The effectiveness of a professionally led support group for men with prostate cancer. *Urologic Nursing, 17*(2), 58–66.

Griffin, A. S., & O'Rourke, M. E. (1999). Not every prostate cancer needs to be treated: The place for expectant management. *North Carolina Medical Journal, 60*(5), 261–267.

Griffiths, T. R. L., & Neal, D. E. (1997). Localized prostate cancer: Early intervention or expectant therapy? *Journal of the Royal Society of Medicine, 90,* 665–669.

Grover, S. A., Coupal, L., Zowall, H., Rajan, R., Trachtenberg, J., Elhilali, M., Chetner, M., & Goldenberg, L. (2000). The clinical burden of prostate cancer in Canada: Forecasts from the Montreal Prostate Cancer Model. *CMAJ, 162,* 977–983.

Guilloneau, B., & Vallancien, G. (2000). Laparoscopic radical prostatectomy: The Montsouris experience. *Journal of Urology, 163*(2), 418–422.

Haas, C. A., & Resnick, M. I. (2000). Trends in diagnosis, biopsy, and imaging. In E. A. Klein (Ed.), *Management of Prostate Cancer* (pp. 87–101). Totowa, NJ: Humana Press.

Haas, G. P., & Sakr, W. A. (1997). Epidemiology of prostate cancer. *CA: Cancer Journal for Clinicians, 47,* 273–287.

Haberman, M. (1995). The meaning of cancer therapy: Bone marrow transplantation as an exemplar of therapy. *Seminars in Oncology Nursing, 11,* 23–31.

Hanks, G. E. (2000). Conformal radiotherapy for prostate cancer. *Annals of Medicine, 32*(1), 57–63.

Hanks, G. E., & Horowitz, E. M. (2000). External beam radiation therapy for prostate cancer. *CA: A Cancer Journal for Clinicians, 50*(6), 349–375.

Hanlon, A. L., Bruner, D. W., Peter, P., & Hanks, G. E. (2001). Quality of life study in prostate cancer patients treated with three-dimensional conformal radiation therapy: Comparing late bowel and bladder quality of life symptoms to that of the normal population. *International Journal of Radiation Oncology, Biology & Physics, 49*(1), 51–59.

Hardman, A., Maguire, P., & Crowther, D. (1989). The recognition of psychiatric morbidity on a medical oncology ward. *J of Psychosom Res, 33,* 235–239.

Harris, J. L. (1997). Treatment of postprostatectomy urinary incontinence with behavioral methods. *Clinical Nurse Specialist, 11*(4), 159–166.

Harrison, L. (2000). Radiation therapy and anemia: Magnitude of the problem. In *Oncology treatment updates.* Medscape, Inc.

Healey, J. H., & Brown, H. K. (1997). Complications of bone metastases. *Cancer, Supplement, 88*(12), 2940–2951.

Heinonen, O. P., Albanes, D., Virtamo, J., Taylor, P. R., Huttunen, J. K., Hartman, A. M., Haapakoski, J., Malila, N., Rautalahti, M., Ripatti, S., Maenpaa, H., Teerenhovi, L., Koss, L., Virolainen, M., & Edwards, B. K. (1998). Prostate cancer and supplementation with alpha-tocopherol and beta-carotene: Incidence and mortality in a controlled trial. *Journal of the National Cancer Institute, 90,* 440–446.

Held, J. L., Osborne, D. M., Volpe, H., & Waldman, R. (1994). Cancer of the prostate: Treatment and nursing implications. *Oncology Nursing Forum, 21,* 1517–1529.

Held-Warmkessel, J. (2000). Chemotherapy for prostate cancer. In J. Held-Warmkessel (Ed.), *Contemporary issues in prostate cancer* (pp. 195–226). Sudbury, MA: Jones and Bartlett Publishers.

Held-Warmkessel, J. (2000). Prostate Cancer. In C. N. Yarbro, M. H. Frogge, M. Goodman, & S. L. Gtoenwald, *Cancer Nursing: Principles and practice* (7th ed., chapter 64; pp. 1427–1451). Sudbury, MA: Jones and Bartlett.

Hewitt, A. (2001). Early catheter removal following radical perineal prostatectomy: A randomized clinical trial. *Urologic Nursing, 21*(1), 37–38.

Heyman, E. N., & Rosner, T. T. (1996). Prostate cancer: An intimate view from patients and their spouses. *Urologic Nursing, 16*(2), 37–44.

Hilderley, L. J. (1992). Pain and fatigue. In K. H. Dow & L. J. Hilderley (Eds.), *Nursing care in radiation oncology.* Philadelphia: Saunders.

Hilderley, L., & Dow, K. H. (1991). Radiation oncology. In S. Baird, R.

McCorkle, & M. Grant (Eds.), *Cancer nursing: A comprehensive textbook*. Philadelphia: Saunders.

Hillman, J. L., & Stricker, G. (1994). A linkage of knowledge and attitudes toward elderly sexuality: Not necessarily a uniform relationship. *The Gerontologist, 34,* 256–260.

Hodge, K. K., McNeal, J. E., & Stamey, T. E. (1989). Ultrasound guided transrectal core biopsies of the palpable abnormal prostate. *Journal of Urology, 142,* 66.

Holland, J. C., & Lewis, S. (2000). *The human side of cancer: Living with hope, coping with uncertainty.* New York: HarperCollins Publishers.

Holm, H. H., Juul, N., Pedersen, J. F., Hansen, H., & Stroyer, J. (1983). Transperineal iodine-125 seed implantation in prostate cancer guided by transrectal ultrasonography. *Journal of Urology, 130,* 283–286.

Holmes, B. (1987). Psychological evaluation and preparation of patient and family. *Cancer, 60,* 2121–2024.

Horowitz, M., Wilner, N., & Alvarez, W. (1979). Impact of event scale: A measure of subjective stress. *Psychosomatic Medicine, 41,* 209–218.

Hortobagyi, G. N., Theriault, R., Porter, L., Blayney, D., Lipton, A., Sinoff, C., Wheeler, H., Simeone, J. F., Seaman, J., Knight, R. D., Heffernan, M., & Reitsma, D. (1996). Efficacy of pamidronate in reducing skeletal complications in patients with breast cancer and lytic bone metastases. *New Eng J Med. 335*(24), 1785–1791.

Hudson, R. (1999). Brachytherapy treatments increasing among Medicare population. *Health Policy Brief of the American Urologic Association, 9,* 1.

Huggins, C., Stevens, R. E., & Hodges, C. V. (1941). Studies on prostate cancer: Effect of castration on advanced carcinoma of the prostate gland. *Archives of Surgery 1941, 43,* 209.

International Agency for Research on Cancer (1982). *The rubber industry.* International Agency for Research on Cancer monograph on evaluating carcinogenic risk in chemical manufacturing, 28, 1486.

International Union Against Cancer (1992). Urological tumors: Prostate. In P. Hermanek & L. H. Sobin (Eds.), *TNM classification of malignant tumors* (4th ed., pp. 141–144). Berlin: Springer-Verlag.

Iverson, P., Tyrrell, C. J., Kaisary, A. V., Anderson, J. B., Van Poppel, H., Tammela, T. L., Chamberlain, M., Carroll, K., & Melezinek, I. (2000). Bicalutamide monotherapy compared with castration in patients with nonmetastatic locally advanced prostate cancer: 6. 3 years of follow up. *Journal of Urology, 164*(5), 1579–1582.

Jacob, F., Salomon, L., Hoznek, A., Antiphon, P., Chopin, D. K., & Abbou, C. C. (2000). Laporoscopic radical prostatectomy: Preliminary results. *European Urology, 37*(5), 615–620.

Jacobson, V. R., Grann, A. I., Neuget, A., Flug, S., Gorin S. Sheinfeld,

Klaus, L., Benson, M. C., & Petrylak, D. L. (1999). Use of complementary/alternative medicine among prostate cancer patients. Abstract #1228. Proceedings from the 35th Annual Meeting American Society of Clinical Oncology.

Jacox, A., Carr, D. B., Payne, R., et al. (1994, March). Management of cancer pain. Clinical Practice Guideline No 9. AHCPR Publication No 94-0592. Rockville, MD. Agency for Health Care Policy and Research, U. S. Department of Health and Human Services, Public Health Service.

Janknegt, R. A. (1993). Total androgen blockade with the use of orchiectomy and nilutamide (Anandron) or placebo as treatment of metastatic prostate cancer. *Anandron International Study Group Cancer, 72*(12 Suppl), 3874–3877.

Jarvis, C. (2000). *Physical examination and health assessment.* Philadelphia: Saunders.

Jenkinson, J., Wilson-Pawels, L., Jewett, M. A. S., & Woolridge, N. (1998). Development of a hypermedia program to assist patients with localized prostate cancer in making treatment decisions. *Journal of Biocommunication, 25*(2), 2–11.

Jewett, H. J. (1975). The present status of radical prostatectomy for stages A and B prostatic cancer. *Urologic Clinics of North America, 2*(1), 105–24

Johansson, J. E., Adami, H. O., Andersson, S. O., Bergstrom, R., Holmberg, L., & Krusemo, U. B. (1992). High 10-year survival rate in patients with early, untreated prostatic cancer. *Journal of the American Medical Association, 267,* 2191–2196.

Johnson, B. L. (1998). Prevention and early detection. In B. L. Johnson & J. Gross (Eds.), *Handbook of oncology nursing* (3rd ed., pp. 241–262). Sudbury, MA: Jones and Bartlett.

Joly, F., Brune, D., Coulette, J. E., Lesasunier, F., Penny, J. et al. (1998). Health related quality of life and sequelae in patients treated with brachytherapy and external beam irradiation for localized prostate cancer. *Annals of Oncology, 9,* 751–757.

Joranson, D. E., Cleeland, C. S., Weissman, D. E., & Gilson, A. M. (1992). Opioids for cancer and non-cancer pain: A survey of state medical board members. *Fed Bull, 79,* 15–49.

Joseph, A. C. (2001). Male pelvic anatomy/post-prostatectomy incontinence. *Urologic Nursing, 21*(1), 25–27.

Kain, C. D., Reilly, N., & Schultz, E. D. (1990). The older adult: A comparative assessment. *Nursing Clinics of North America, 25,* 833–848.

Kamradt, J. M., & Pienta, K. J. (2000). Prostate cancer chemotherapy. In L. W. K. Chung, W. B. Isaacs, & J. W. Simons (Eds.), *Prostate cancer: Biology, genetics, and the new therapeutics* (pp. 415–431). Totowa, NJ: Humana Press Inc.

Kamradt, J. M., & Pienta, K. J. (2000). New paradigms in the management of hormone refractory disease. In E. A. Klein (Ed.), *Management of prostate cancer* (pp. 289–303). Totowa, NJ: Humana Press, Inc.

Kaplan, H. S (1990). Sex, intimacy and the aging process. *Journal of theAmerican Academy of Psychoanalysis,* 185–205.

Kassabian, V., & Graham, S. (1995). Urologic and male genital cancers. In G. Murphy, W. Lawrence, & R. Lenhard (Eds.), *American cancer society textbook of clinical oncology.* Atlanta, GA: The American Cancer Society.

Kelly, L. D. (1999). Nursing assessment and patient management. *Seminars in Oncology Nursing, 15*(4), 282–291.

King, K. G., Nail, L. M., Kreamer, K., Strohl, R. A., & Johnson, J. E. (1985). Patients' descriptions of the experience receiving radiation therapy. *Oncology Nursing Forum, 12*(4), 55–61.

Kiningham, B. B. (1998). Physical activity and the primary prevention of cancer. *Primary Care: Clinics in Office Practice, 25*(2), 515–536.

King, C., Haberman, M., Berry, D. Bush, N., Butler, N., Dow, K. H., Ferrell, B., Grant, M., Gue, D., Hinds, P., Kreuer, J., Padilla, G., Underwood, S. (1997). Quality of life and the cancer experience: The state of the knowledge. *Oncology Nursing Forum, 24*(1), 27–42.

Kinney, M., Burfitt, S., Stullenbarger, E., Rees, B., DeBolt, M. (1996). Quality of life in cardiac patient research: A meta-analysis. *Nursing Research, 45*(3), 173–80.

Kissane, D. W., Block S., McKenzie M., McDowell AC., Nitzan, R. (1998). Family grief therapy: A preliminary account of a new model to promote healthy family functioning during palliative care and bereavement. *Psychooncology, 7*(1), 14–25.

Klimaszewski, A. D., & Karlowicz, K. A. (1995). Cancer of the male genitalia. In K. A. Karlowicz (Ed.), *Urologic nursing principles and practice* (pp. 271–308). Philadelphia, PA: Saunders.

Klotz, L. (2000). Hormone therapy for patients with prostate carcinoma. *Cancer 2000 Jun 15, 88*(12 Suppl), 3009–3014.

Koppie, T. M., Grossfeld, G. D., Miller, D., Yu, J., Stier, D., Broering, J. M., Lubeck, D., Henning, J. M., Flanders, S. C., & Carroll, P. R. (2000). Patterns of treatment of patients with prostate cancer initially managed with surveillance: Results from The CaPSURE database. Cancer of the Prostate Strategic Urological Research Endeavor. *Journal of Urology, 164,* 81–88.

Kornblith, A. B., Herr, H. W., Ofman, U. S., Scher, H. I., & Holland, J. C. (1994). Quality of life of patients with prostate cancer and their spouses. *Cancer, 73,* 2791–2802.

Kramer, B. S., Brown, M. L., Prorok, P. C., Potosky, A., L., & Gohagan, J. K. (1993). Prostate cancer screening: What we know and what we need to know. *Annals of Internal Medicine, 119,* 914–923.

Krishnam, K., Ruffin, M. T., & Brenner, D. E. (1998). Cancer chemoprevention: A new way to treat cancer before it happens. *Primary Care: Clinics in Office Practice, 25*(2), 361–379.

Krishnasamy, M. (2000). Fatigue in advanced cancer—Meaning before measurement? *Int J Nurs Stud, 37*(5), 401–414.

Krizek, C., Roberts, C., Ragan, R., Ferrara, J. J., & Lord, B. (1999). Gender and cancer support group participation. *Cancer Practice, 7*(2), 86–92.

Krupski, T., Petroni G. R., Bissonette, E. A., & Theodorescue, D. (2000). Quality of life comparison of radial prostatectomy and interstitial brachytherapy in the treatment of localized prostate cancer. *Urology, 55,* 736–742.

Kubricht, D. W. (1984). Therapeutic self-care demands expressed by outpatients receiving external radiation therapy. *Cancer Nursing, 7,* 43–52.

Laing, A. H., Ackery, D. M., Bayly, R. J., Buchanan, R. B., Lewington, V. J., McEwan, A. J., Macleod, P. M., & Zivanovic, M. A. (1991). Strontium-89 chloride for pain palliation in prostate skeletal malignancy. *Br J Radiol 64,* 816–822.

Landis, S. H., Murray, T., Bolden, S., & Wingo, P. A. (1999). Cancer statistics 1999. *CA Cancer Journal for Clinicians, 49,* 8–31.

Lassen, P. M., & Kearse, W. S. (1995). Rectal injuries during radical perineal prostatectomy. *Urology, 45*(2), 266–269.

Lawton, C. A., Won, M., Pilepich, M. V., Asbell, S. O., Shipley, W. U., Hanks, G. E., Cox, J. D., Perez, C. A., Sause, W. T., Daggett, S. R. L., & Rubin, P. (1991). Long-term treatment sequelae following external beam irradiation for adenocarcinoma of the prostate: Analysis of RTOG studies 75-06 and 77-06. *International Journal of Radiation Oncology Biology & Physics, 21,* 935–939.

Lee, F., Littrup, P. J., Torp-Pedersen, S. T., Mettlin, C., McHugh, T. A., Gray, J. M., Kumasaka, G. H., & Mcleaary, R. D. (1988). Prostate cancer: Comparison of transrectal U.S. and digital rectal examination for screening, *Radiology, 168,* 389–394.

Lee, N., Wuu, C., Brody, R., Laguna, J. L., Katz, A. E., Bagiella, E., & Ennis, R. D. (2000). Factors predicting for postimplantation urinary retention after permanent prostate brachytherapy. *International Journal of Radiation Oncology Biology & Physics, 48*(5), 1457–1460.

Lee, W. R., Schultheisis, T. E., Hanlon, A. L., Hanks, G. E. . (1996). Urinary incontinence following external beam radiotherapy for clinically localized prostate cancer. *Urology, 48,* 95–99.

Lewington, V. J., McEwain, A. J. B., Ackery, D. M., Bayly, R. J., Keeling, D. H., Macleod, P. M., Porter, A. T., & Zivanovic, M. A. (1991). A prospective randomized double-blind crossover study to examine

the efficacy of strontium-89 in pain palliation in patients with advanced prostate cancer metastatic to bone. *Eur J Cancer, 27,* 954–958.
Lewis, J. H. (2000). The role of the NP in the diagnosis and management of erectile dysfunction. *The Nurse Practitioner, 25*(6), 14–18.
Lim, A., Brandon, A., Fiedler, J., Brickman, A., Boyer, C., Raub, W., Jr, Soloway, M. (1995). Quality of life: Radical prostatectomy versus radiation therapy for prostate cancer. *Journal of Urology, 154*(4), 1420–1425.
Lind, J., Kravitz, K., & Greig, B. (1993). Urologic and male genital malignancies. In S. Groenwald, M. Frogge, M. Goodman, & C. H. Yarbro (Eds.), *Cancer nursing: Principles & practice* (pp. 1258–1279). Boston: Jones & Bartlett.
Lindeman, C. A. (1988). Patient education: Part II. *Annual Review of Nursing Research, 6,* 199–212
Lipowski Z. (1990). Delirium in geriatric patients. In *Delirium: Acute confusional states* (pp. 413–441). New York: Oxford University Press.
Littrup, P. J., Lee, F., & Mettlin, C. J. (1992). Prostate cancer screening: Current trends and future implications. *CA Cancer Journal for Clinicians, 42,* 198–211.
Litwin, M. S. (1994). Measuring health related quality of life in men with prostate cancer. *The Journal of Urology, 152,* 1882–1887.
Litwin, M. S., Flanders, S. C., Pasta, D. J., Stoddard, M. L., Lubeck, D. P., & Henning, J. M. (1999). Sexual function and bother after radical prostatectomy or radiation for prostate cancer: Multivariate quality-of-life analysis from CaPSURE. Cancer of the Prostate Strategic Urologic Research Endeavor. *Urology, 54*(3), 503–508.
Litwin, M. S., Hays, R. D., Fink, A. Ganz, P. A., Leake, B, Leach, G. E., & Brook, R. H. (1995). Quality of life outcomes in men treated for localized prostate cancer. *Journal of the American Medical Association, 273,* 129–135.
Litwin, M. S., Hays, R. D., Ganz, P. A., Leake, B., & Brook, R. H. (1998). The UCLA prostate cancer index: Development, reliability and validity of a health related quality of life measure. *Medical Care, 36,* 1002–1012.
Litwin, M., & McGuigan, K. (1999). Accuracy of recall in health-related quality-of-life assessment among men treated for prostate cancer. *Journal of Clinical Oncology, 17*(9), 2882–2888.
Loescher, L. J. (1997). Dynamics of cancer prevention. In S. L. Groenwald, M. H. Frogge, M. Goodman, & C. H. Yarbro (Eds.), *Cancer Nursing: Principles and Practice* (4th ed., pp. 94–107). Sudbury, MA: Jones and Bartlett.
Lubke, W. L., Optenberg, S. A., & Thompson, I. M. (1994). Analysis of

the first-year cost of a prostate cancer screening and treatment program in the United States. *Journal of National Cancer Institute, 86,* 1790–1792.

Ludwig, H., & Fritz, E. (1998). Anemia in cancer patients. *Seminars in Oncology, 25,* 2–6.

Lund-Nilsen, T. I., Johnson, R., & Vatten, L. J. (2000). Socioeconomic and lifestyle factors associated with the risk of prostate cancer. *British Journal of Cancer, 82*(7), 1358–1363.

MacCormick, R. E., & Mackinnon, K. J. (1990). Decision making in cancer treatment: Age and socio-economic status as independent variables. *Medical Teacher, 12,* 353–355.

Maher, K. E. (1996). Late effects of radiation therapy: Quality of life. Cope, 4–7.

Mahon, S. M., & Casperson, D. M. (1997). Exploring the psychosocial meaning of recurrent cancer: A descriptive study. *Cancer Nursing, 20*(3), 178–186.

Mahon, S. M., Casperson, D., & Wozniak-Petrofsky, J. (1990). Prostate cancer: Screening through treatment and nursing implications. *Urology Nursing,* 5–1.

Mahon, S. M. (2000). The role of the nurse in developing cancer screening programs. *Oncology Nursing Forum, 27*(Suppl. 9), 19–27.

Mannix, K., Ahmedzai, S. H., & Anderson, H. (2000). Using bisphosphonates to control the pain of bone metastases: Evidence-based guidelines for palliative care. *Palliative Med, 14,* 455–461.

Mantz, C. A., Song, P., Farhangi, E., Nautiyal, J., Awan, J., Ignacio, L., Weichselbaum, R., & Vijayakumar, S. (1997). Potency probability following conformal megavoltage radiotherapy using conventional doses for localized prostate cancer. *International Journal of Radiation Oncology, Biology & Physics, 37*(3), 551–557.

Marschke, P. (2000). Measurement of urinary continence recovery following radical prostatectomy. In M. T. Nolan, & V. Mock (Eds.), *Measuring patient outcomes* (pp. 185–195). Thousand Oaks, CA. Sage Publication.

Massie, M. J., & Holland, J. C. (1992). The cancer patient with pain: Psychiatric complications and their management. *J Pain Symptom Manage, 7,* 99–109

Mazur, D. J., & Hickam, D. H. (1996). Patient preferences for management of localized prostate cancer. *Western Journal of Medicine, 165,* 26–30.

Mazur, D. J., & Merz, J. F. (1995). Older male patients' willingness to trade off urologic adverse outcomes for a better chance at 5-year survival in the clinical setting of prostate cancer. *Journal of the American Geriatrics Society, 43,* 979–984.

Mazur, D. J., Hickam, D. H., & Mazur, M. D. (1999). How patients' preferences for medical information influence treatment choice in a case of high risk and high uncertainty: Asymptomatic localized prostate cancer. *Medical Decision Making, 19,* 394–398.

McCaffery, M., & Ferrell, B. R. (1992a). Does life-style affect your pain-control decisions? *Nurs, 22*(4), 58–61.

McCaffery, M., & Ferrell, B. R. (1992b). Does the gender gap affect your pain-control decisions? *Nurs, 22*(8), 48–51.

McCaffery, M., & Ferrell, B. R. (1992c). How vital are vital signs? Nurs, 22(1), 42–46.

McCaffery, M., & Ferrell, B. R. (1991). Patient age: Does it affect your pain-control decisions? *Nurs, 21*(9), 44–48.

McCaffery, M., & Ferrell, B. R. (1997). Nurse's knowledge of pain assessment and management: How much progress have we made? *J Pain Sympt Manage, 14,* 175–188.

McDonald, M. V., Passik, S. D., Dugan, W., Rosenfeld, B., Theobald, D. E., & Edgerton, S. (1999). Nurse's recognition of depression in their patients with cancer. *Oncology Nursing Forum, 26*(3), 593–599.

McHale, M. (2000). Cancer-related fatigue: An introduction. *Oncology Issues, 15*(4), supp, 6.

McKee, J. M. (1994). Cues to action in prostate cancer screening. *Oncology Nursing Forum, 21,* 1171–1176.

Meikle, W., & Stanish, W. M. (1982). Familial prostate cancer risk and low testosterone. *Journal of Clinical Endocrine Metabolism, 54,* 1104–1108.

Mannix, K., Ahmedzai, S. H., & Anderson, H. (2000). Using bisphosphonates to control the pain of bone metastases: Evidence-based guidelines for palliative care. *Palliative Med, 14,* 455–461.

Melzack, R., & Katz, J. (1992). The McGill Pain Questionnaire: Appraisal and current status. In D. Turk, & R. Melzack (Eds.), *Handbook of pain assessment* (pp. 152–168). New York: Guilford.

Mendoza, T. R., Wang, X. S., Cleeland, C. S., Morrissey, M., Johnson, B. A., Wendt, J. K., & Huber, S. L. (1999). The rapid assessment of fatigue severity in cancer patients. *Cancer Practice, 85*(5), 1186–1196.

Meniscus. (unknown). As cited in J. Bartlett, *Familiar quotations* (16th ed., p. 79). Boston: Little, Brown and Company.

Meredith, C. E. (1995). Erectile dysfunction. In K. A. Karlowicz (Ed.), *Urologic nursing principles and practice* (pp. 332–359). Philadelphia, PA: Saunders.

Merrick, G. S., Butler, W. M., Dorsey, A. T., Galbreath, R. W., Blatt, H., & Lief, J. H. (2000). Rectal function following prostate brachytherapy. *International Journal of Radiation Oncology Biology & Physics, 48*(3), 667–674.

Merrick, G. S., Butler, W. M., Farthing, W. H., Dorsey, A. T., & Adamovich, E. (1998). The impact of Gleason score accuracy as a criterion for prostate brachytherapy patient selection. *Journal of Brachytherapy International, 14,* 113–121.

Merrick, G. S., Butler, W. M., Lief, J. H., Stipetich, R. L., Abel, L. J., & Dorsey, A. T. (1999). Efficacy of sildenafil citrate in prostate brachytherapy patients with erectile dysfunction. *Urology, 53*(6), 1112–1116.

Mettlin, C., Littrup, P. J., Kane, R. A., Murphy, G. P., Lee, F., Chesley, A., Badalament, R., & Mostofi, F. K. (1994). Relative sensitivity and specificity of serum prostate specific antigen (PSA) level compared with age-referenced PSA, PSA density and PSA change. *Cancer, 74,* 1615–1620.

Michalski, J. M., Purdy, J. A., Winter, K., Roach, M., Vijayakumar, S., Sandler, H. M., Markoe, A. M., Ritter, M. A., Russell, K. J., Sailer, S., Harms, W. B., Perez, C. A., Wilder, R. B., Hanks, G. E., & Cox, J. D. (2000). Preliminary report of toxicity following 3D radiation therapy for prostate cancer on 3DOG/RTOG 9406. *International Journal of Radiation Oncology, Biology & Physics, 46*(2), 391–402.

Mills, P. K. (1999). Review: Nutritional and socioeconomic factors in relation to prostate cancer mortality: A cross-national study. *Journal of the National Cancer Institute, 91*(8), 725–726.

Mills, P. K., Beeson, W. L., Phillips, R. I., & Fraser, G. E. (1989). Cohort study of diet, lifestyle, and prostate cancer in Adventist men. *Cancer, 64,* 598–604.

Mirels, H. (1989). Metastatic disease to long bones. A proposed scoring system for diagnosing impending pathological fractures. *Clin Orthop, 249,* 256–264.

Mishel, M. H. (1988). Uncertainty in illness. *Image, 20,* 225–232.

Mishel, M. (1999). *Uncertainty management intervention.* Paper presented at the Congressional Breakfast Briefing, Friends of the National Institute of Nursing Research, Washington, DC.

Monga, U., Kerrigan, A. J., Thornby, J., & Monga, T. N. (1999). Prospective study of fatigue in localized prostate cancer patients undergoing radiotherapy. *Radiation Oncology Investigations, 7,* 178–185.

Montie, J. E., & Pienta, K. J. (1994). Review of the role of androgenic hormones in the epidemiology of benign prostatic hypertrophy and prostate cancer. *Urology, 43,* 892–899.

Montie, J. E. (2000). Staging systems for prostate cancer. In N. J. Vogelzang, P. T. Scardino, W. U. Shiplet, & D. S. Coffey (Eds.), *Comprehensive textbook of genitourinary oncology* (2nd ed., pp. 673–679). Philadelphia: Lippincott Williams & Wilkins.

Montironi, R., Mazzucchelli, R., Marshall, J. R., & Bartels, P. H. (1999). Prostate cancer prevention: Review of target populations, pathological biomarkers, and chemopreventive agents. *Journal of Clinical Pathology, 52,* 793–803.

Moore, K., & Estey, A. (1999). The early post-operative concerns of men after radical prostatectomy. *Journal of Advanced Nursing, 29*(5), 1121–1129.

Moore, A. R., & O'Keefe, S. T. (1999). Drug-induced cognitive impairment in the elderly. *Drugs Aging, July15*(1), 15–28.

Morgan, T. O., Jacobsen, S. J., McCarthy, W. F., Jacobson, D. J., McLeod, D. G., & Moul, J. W. (1996). Age-specific reference ranges for serum prostate-specific antigen in black men. *The New England Journal of Medicine, 335,* 304–310.

Morra, M. N., & Das, S. (1993). Prostate cancer: Epidemiology and etiology. In S. Das & E. D. Crawford (Eds.), *Cancer of the prostate* (pp. 1–12). New York: Marcel Dekker.

Morra, M. (2000). New opportunities for nurses as patient advocates. *Seminars in Oncology Nursing, 16*(1), 57–64.

Morse, R., & Resnick, M. (1990). Detection of clinically occult prostate cancer. *Urologic Clinics of North America, 17*(3), 567–74.

Morton, R. Jr. (1994). Racial differences in adenocarcinoma of the prostate in North American men. *Urology, 44,* 637–645.

Moul, J. W. (1998). Contemporary hormonal management of advanced prostate cancer. *Oncology, 12*(5), 499–504.

Mundy, G. R. (1997). Mechanisms of bone metastasis. *Cancer Supplement. 80/8.* 1546–1556.

Nag, S., Beyer, D., Friedland, J., Grimm, P., & Nath, R. (1999). American brachytherapy society (ABS) recommendations for transperineal permanent brachytherapy of prostate cancer. *International Journal of Radiation Oncology, Biology & Physics, 44*(4), 789–799.

Nail, L. M., & King, K. B. (1987). Fatigue. *Seminars in Oncology Nursing, 3*(4), 257–262.

Naitoh, J., Zeiner, R. L., & Dekernion, J. B. (1998). Diagnosis and treatment of prostate cancer. *American Family Physician, 57,* 1531–1539.

Nam, R. K., Klotz, L. H., Jewett, MA., Danjoux, C., & Trachtenberg, J. (1998). Prostate specific antigen velocity as a measure of the natural history of prostate cancer: Defining a "rapid riser" subset. *British Journal of Urology, 81,* 100–104.

Narayan, P. (1995). Neoplasms of the prostate gland. In E. Tanagoho & J. McAninch (Eds.), *Smith's general urology* (14th ed., pp. 392–433). Norwalk, CT: Appleton & Lange.

Nath, R., Meigooni, A. S., & Melillo, A. (1992). Some treatment planning considerations for 103-Pd and 125-I permanent interstitial implants. *International Journal of Radiation Oncology Biology & Physics, 22,* 1131–1138.

National Comprehensive Cancer Networks (NCCN). (1997). Update of the NCCN guidelines for treatment of prostate cancer. *Oncology, 11*(11A), 180–193.

National Comprehensive Center Networks. NCCN Prostate Cancer Guidelines. [on-line]. Available: www. nccn. org.

National Institutes of Health Consensus Development Panel. (1988). Consensus Statement: The management of clinically localized prostate cancer. *NCI Monogram, 7,* 3–6.

Neulander, E. Z., Duncan, R. C., Tiguert, R., Posey, J. T., & Soloway, M. S. (2000). Deferred treatment of localized prostate cancer in the elderly: The impact of the age and stage at the time of diagnosis on the treatment decision. *Bju International, 85,* 699–704.

Newman, M. L., Brennan, M., & Passik, S. (1996). Lymphedema complicated by pain & psychological distress: A case with complex treatment needs. *J Pain Symptom Manage, 12,* 376–379.

Newschaffer, C. (1997). The impact of co-morbidity on life expectancy among men with localized prostate cancer. *Journal of Urology, 157*(3), 964–965.

Newton, M., & Hannay, J. (1998). Nonsteroidal anti-androgens: Role in treating advanced prostate cancer. *Urologic Nursing, 18*(1), 56–83.

Ng, K., & von Guten, C. F. (1998). Symptoms and attitudes of 100 consecutive patients admitted to an acute hospice/palliative care unit. *J Pain Sympt Manag. 16,* 307–316.

Nightengale, B., Brune, M., Blizzard, S., Ashley-Johnson, M., & Slan, S. (1995). Strontium chloride sr^{89} for treating pain from metastatic bone disease. *Am J Health—Syst Pharm, 52,* 2189–2195.

Norrish, A. E., Ferguson, L. R., Knize, M. G., Felton, J. S., Sharpe, S. J., & Jackson, R. (1999). Heterocyclic amine content of cooked meat and the risk of prostate cancer. *Journal of the National Cancer Institute, 91*(23), 2038–2044.

Norrish, A. E., Jackson, R. T., Sharpe, S. J., & Skeaff, C. M. (2000). Prostate cancer and dietary carotenoids. *American Journal of Epidemiology, 151*(2), 119–123.

Oesterling, J. E., Jacobsen, S. J., Chute, C. G., Guess, H. A., Girman, C. J., Panser, L. A., & Lieber, M. M. (1993). Serum prostate-specific antigen in a community-based population of healthy men. *Journal of the American Medical Association, 270,* 860–864.

Oesterling, J. E., Martin, S., Bergstralh, E., & Lowe, F. (1993). The use of prostate-specific antigen in staging patients with newly diagnosed prostate cancer. *Journal of the American Medical Association, 269,* 57–60.

Ojdeby, Claezon, Brekkan, Haggman, & Nolan (1996). Urinary incontinence and sexual impotence after radical prostatectomy. *Scandinavian Journal of Urologic Nephrology, 30*(6), 473–477.

Oleson, M. (1990). Subjectively perceived quality of life. *Image, 22,* 187–190.

Olivotto, I., Gelmon, K., & Kuusk, U. (1996). *Intelligent patients guide to breast cancer.* Vancouver: Intelligent Patient Guide.

Olsen, S. J., Morrison, C. H., & Ashley, B. W. (1998). Prevention of cancer. In J. K. Itano & K. N. Taoka (Eds.), Core Curriculum for Oncology Nursing (3rd ed., pp. 681–694). Philadelphia: Saunders.

Oncology Nursing Society/American Nurse's Association. (1996). Statement of the scope and standards of oncology nursing practice. Washington, DC: American Nurses Publishing.

Orenstein, R., & Wong, E. S. (1999). Urinary tract infections in adults. *American Family Physician, 59*(5), 1225–1234.

O'Rourke, M. E. (1997). Prostate cancer treatment selection: The family decision process. Unpublished dissertation, University of North Carolina, Chapel Hill.

O'Rourke, M. E., & Germino, B. B. (1998). Prostate cancer treatment selection: A focus group exploration. *Oncology Nursing Forum, 25,* 97–103.

O'Rourke, M. E., (1999). Narrowing the options: The process of deciding on prostate cancer treatment. *Cancer Investigation, 17,* 349–359.

Padilla, G., Ferrell, B., Grant, M., & Rhiner, M. (1990). Defining the content domain of quality of life for cancer patients with pain. *Cancer Nursing, 13*(2), 108–115.

Padilla, G., Grant, M., Ferrell, B., & Presant, C. (1996). Quality of life—cancer. In B. Spilker (Ed.) *Quality of life and pharmacoeconomics in clinical trials.* Philadelphia: Lippincott-Raven Publishers.

Padma-Nathan, H., & Forrest, C. (2000). Diagnosis and treatment of erectile dysfunction: The process of care model. *The Nurse Practitioner, 25*(6), 4–10.

Palmer, J. S., & Chodak, G. W. (1996). Defining the role of surveillance in management of localized prostate cancer. *The Urolgic Clinics of North America, 23,* 551–556.

Palmer, M., Powel, L., & Somerfield, M. (1999). Coping with urinary incontinence after prostate cancer surgery. Unpublished data.

Pappas P, Stravodimos KG, Mitropoulos D, Kontopoulou C, Haramogolis S, Giannopoulou M, Tzortzis G & Giannopoulos A. (2000). Role of percutaneous urinary diversion in malignant and benign obstructive uropathy. *J Endourol 14,* 401–405.

Parker, S. L., Davis, K. J., Wingo, P. A., Reise, L. A., Heath, C. W. Jr (1998). Cancer statistics by race and ethnicity. *CA: Cancer Journal for Clinicians, 48,* 31–38

Parkin, D., Pisani, P., & Ferlay, J. (1999). Global cancer statistics. *CA: A Cancer Journal for Clinicians, 49*(1), 33–64.

Partin, A. W., Kattan, M. W., Subong, E. N., Walsh, P. C., Wojno, K. J., Oesterling, J. E., Scardino, P. T., & Pearson, J. D. (1997). Combination of prostate-specific antigen, clinical stage, and Gleason Score to predict pathological stage of localized prostate cancer: A multi-institutional update. *Journal of the American Medical Association, 277*(2), 1445–1451.

Pasero, C., Gordon, D. B., McCaffery, M., & Ferrell, B. R. (1999). Building An insitutional commitment to improving pain management. In M. McCaffery & C Pasero (Eds.), *Pain Clinical Manual* (2nd ed.). St. Louis, MO: Mosby.

Passik, S. D., Dugan, W., McDonald, M. V., Rosenfeld, B., Theobald, D., & Edgerton, S. (1998). Oncologists' recognition of depression in their patients with cancer. *J Clin Oncol, 16,* 1594–1600.

Passik, S., Newman, M., Brennan, M., & Holland, J. (1993). Psychiatric consultation for women undergoing rehabilitation for upper-extremity lymphedema following breast cancer treatment. *J Pain Symptom Manage, 8,* 226–233.

Paul, A. B., Love, C., & Chisholm, G. D. (1994). The management of bilateral ureteric obstruction and renal failure in advanced prostate cancer. *Br J Urol, 74*(5), 642–645.

Payne, D. K., & Massie, M. J. (2000). Anxiety in palliative care. In H. M. Chochinov & W. Breitbart (Eds.), *Handbook of psychiatry in palliative medicine* (pp. 63–74). New York: Oxford University Press.

Pereira, J., Mancini, I., & Walker, P. (1998). The role of bisphosphonates in malignant bone pain: A review. *Jour Palliative Care, 14,* 25–36.

Perez, C. A. (1998). Prostate. In C. A. Perez & L. W. Brady (Eds.), *Principles and practices of radiation oncology* (3rd ed.). Philadelphia: Lippincott-Raven Publishers.

Perez, C. A., Michalski, J. M., Purdy, J. A., Wasserman, T. H., Williams, K., & Lockett, M. A. (2000). Three-dimensional conformal therapy or standard irradiation in localized carcinoma of prostate: Preliminary results of a nonrandomized comparison. *International Journal of Radiation Oncology Biology & Physics, 47*(3), 629–637.

Peschel, R. E. (1990). External beam versus interstitial implant therapy for prostate cancer: A review. *Endocurietherapy/Hypertheria Oncology, 6,* 231–237.

Peschel, R. E. (1997). External-beam radiation therapy for local prostate cancer. In M. S. Ernstoff, J. A. Heaney, & R. E. Peschel (Eds.), *Urologic Cancer.* Cambridge: Blackwell Science.

Petrek JA, Pressman PI & Smith RA. (2000). Lymphedema: Current Issues in Research and Management. *CA Cancer J Clin, 50,* 292–307.

Pienta, K., & Esper, P. (1993). Risk factors for prostate cancer. *Annals of Internal Medicine, 118,* 793–802.

Pierce, P. (1993). Deciding on breast cancer treatment: A description of decision behavior. *Nursing Research, 42,* 22–28.

Pilepich, M. V., Asbell, S. O., Mulholland, G. S., & Pajak. T. (1984). Surgical staging in carcinoma of the prostate: The RTOG experience. Radiation Oncology Group. *Prostate, 5,* 471–476.

Pilepich, M. V., Krall, J. M., al-Sarraf, M., John, M. J., Doggett, R. L., Sause, W. T., Lawton, C. A., Abrams, R. A., Rotman, M., & Rubin, P. (1995). Androgen-deprivation with radiation therapy compared with radiation therapy alone for locally advanced prostate carcinoma: A randomized comparative trial of the radiation therapy oncology group. *Urology, 45,* 616.

Pilepich, M. V., Walz, B. J., & Baglan, R. J. (1987). Postoperative radiation in carcinoma of the prostate. *International Journal of Radiation Oncology Biology & Physics, 10,* 1869–1873.

Piper, B. F., Burke, M. D., Messner, C. M., et al. (Eds.). (1991). Dimensions of caring-taking control of fatigue (monograph) Cleveland, OH: Pro Ed Communication.

Piper, B. F., Lindsey, A. M., Dodd, M. J., Ferketich, S., Paul, S. M., & Weller, S. (1989). The development of an instrument to measure the subjective dimension of fatigue. In S. G. Funk, E. M. Tournquist, M. T. Champagne, L. A. Copp, & R. A. Weise (Eds.), *Key aspects of comfort: Management of pain, fatigue, and nausea.* New York: Springer Publishing.

Pobursky, J. (1995). Prostate cancer: Detection and treatment options. *Todays Or-Nurse, 17,* 5–9.

Popp, B., & Portenoy, R. K. (1996). Management of Chronic Pain in the Elderly. *Pain in the elderly: A report of the task force on pain in the elderly.* Seattle, WA: International Association for the Study of Pain.

Portenoy, R. K., Payne, D., & Jacobsen, P. (1999). Breakthrough pain: Characteristics and impact in patients with cancer pain. *Pain, 81,* 129–134.

Porter, A. T., McEvan, A. J. B., Powe, J. E., Powe, J. E., Reid, R., McGowen, D. G., Lukka, H., Sathyanarayana, J. R., Yakemchuk, V. N., Thomas, G. M., Erlich, L. E., Crook, J., Gulenchyn, K. Y., Hong, K. E., Wesolowski, C., & Yardley, J. (1993). Results of a randomized Phase III trial to evaluate the efficacy of strontium-89 adjuvant to local field external beam irradiation in the management of endocrine resistant metastatic prostate cancer. *Int J Radiati Oncol Biol Phys, 25,* 805–813.

Potosky, A. L., Legler, J., Albertsen, P. C., Stanford, J. L., Gilliand, F. D., Hamilton, A. S., Eley, J. W., Stephenson, R. A., & Harlan, L. C.

(2000). Health outcomes after prostatectomy or radiotherapy for prostate cancer: Results from the Prostate Cancer Outcomes Study. *Journal of the National Cancer Institute, 92,* 1582–1592.

Pound, C. R., Partin, A. W., Eisenberger, M. A., Chan, D. W., Pearson, J. D., & Walsh, P. C. (1999). Natural history of progression after PSA elevation following radical prostatectomy. *Journal of the American Medical Association, 281*(17) 1591–1597.

Powe, B. D. (1996). Cancer fatalism among African Americans: A review of the literature. *Nursing Outlook, 44,* 18–21.

Quilty, P. M., Kirk, D., Bolger, J. J., Dearnaley, D. P., Lewington, V. J., Mason, M. D., Reed, N. S., Russell, J. M., & Yardley, J. (1994). A comparison of the palliative effects of strontium-89 and external beam radiotherapy in metastatic prostatic cancer. *Radiother Oncol, 31,* 33–40.

Quinlan, D., Epstein, J., & Carter, B. (1991). Sexual function following radical prostatectomy: Influence of preservation of neurovascular bundles. *The Journal of Urology, 145*(5), 998–1002.

Rabbani, F., Stapleton, A. M., & Kattan, M. W. (2000). Factors predicting recovery of erections after radical prostatectomy. *Journal of Urology, 164*(6), 1929–1934

Ragde, H., Blasko, J. C., Grimm, P. D., Kenny, G. M., Sylvester, J. E., Hoak, D. C., Landin, K., & Cavanagh, W. (1997). Interstitial iodine-125 radiation without adjuvant therapy in the treatment of clinically localized prostate carcinoma. *Cancer, 80*(3), 442–453.

Ragde, H., Grado, G. L., Nadir, B., & Elgamal, A. A. (2000). Modern prostate brachytherapy. *CA-A Cancer Journal for Clinicians, 50*(6), 380–393.

Ragde, H., & Korb, L. (2000). Brachytherapy for clinically localized prostate cancer. *Seminars in Surgical Oncology, 18,* 45–51.

Reust, C. E., & Mattingly, S. (1996). Family involvement in medical decision making. *Family Medicine, 28*(1), 39–45.

Richardson, A. (1995). Fatigue in cancer patients: A review of the literature. *European Journal of Cancer Care, 4,* 20–32.

Roach, M., Chinn, D. M., Holland, J., & Clarke, M. (1996). A pilot study of sexual function and quality of life following 3D conformal radiotherapy for clinically localized prostate cancer. *International Journal of Radiation Oncology, Biology & Physics, 35*(5), 869–874.

Robinson, D., Pierce, K., Preisser, J., Dugan, E., Suggs, P., & Cohen, S. (1998). Relationship between patient reports of urinary incontinence symptoms and quality of life measures. *Obstetrics & Gynecology, 91,* 224–228.

Rogers, M. J., Watts, D. J., & Russell, R. G. G. (1997). Overview of bisphosphonates. *Cancer Supplement 80*(8), 1652–1660

Roscow, I. (1981). Coalitions in geriatric medicine. In M. Haug (Ed.), *Elderly patients and their doctors.* New York: Spinger Publishing.

Roth, A. J., & Breitbart, W. (1996), Psychiatric emergencies in terminally ill cancer patients. *Hematology/Oncology Clinics of North America: Pain & Palliative Care, 10,* 235–259.

Roth, A. J., Kornblith, A. B., Batel-Copel, L., Peabody, E., Scher, H. I., & Holland, J. C. (1998). Rapid screening for psychologic distress in men with prostate carcinoma. *Cancer, 82,* 1904–1908.

Roth, S. H. (1989). Merits and liabilities of NSAID therapy. *Rheum Dis Clin North Amer, 15,* 479.

Sakr, W. A., Haas, G. P., Cassin, B. F., Pontes, J. E., & Crissman, J. D. (1993). The frequency of carcinoma and intraepithelial neoplasia of the prostate in young males. *Journal of Urology, 150,* 379–385.

Salzman, C. (1991). Geriatric psychopharmacology. In A. Gelenberg, E. L. Bassuck, & S. C. Schoonover (Eds.), *The practitioner's guide to psychoactive drugs* (pp. 319–339). New York: Plenum Medical Book Company.

Santis, W. F., Hoffman, M. A., & DeWolf, W. C. (2000). Early catheter removal in 100 consecutive patients undergoing retropubic prostatectomy. *British Journal of Urology, 85*(9), 1067–1068.

Sartorius, N. (1989). Crossi-cultural comparisons of data about quality of life: A sample of issues, In N. K. Aaronson, & J. Beckmann (Eds.), *The quality of life of cancer patients.* New York: Raven.

Saunders, C. (1989). Pain and imprending death. In P. D. Wall, & R. Melzack (Eds.), *Textbook of pain.* Edinburgh: Churchill Livingston.

Schag, C., Ganz, P., & Heinrich, R. (1991). Cancer Rehabilitation Evaluation System—short form (CARES-SF). A cancer specific rehabilitation and quality of life instrument. *Cancer, 68*(6), 1406–1413.

Scher, H., Isaacs, J., Fuks, Z., & Walsh, P. (1995). Prostate. In M. Abeloff, J. Armitage, A. Lichter, & J. Niederhuber (Eds.), *Clinical oncology.* New York: Churchill-Livingstone.

Schipper, H., Clinch, J., McMurray, A., & Levitt, M. (1984). Measuring the quality of life of cancer patients: The functional living index-cancer: Development and validation. *Journal of Clinical Oncology, 2,* 472–483.

Schover, L. R., von Eschenbach, A. C., Smith, D. B., & Gonzalez, J. (1984). Sexual rehabilitation of urologic patients: A practical approach. *CA: A Cancer Journal for Clinicians, 34*(2), 3–11

Schroder, F. H. (1994). The European Screening Study for prostate cancer. *Canadian Journal of Oncology, 4*(Suppl 1), 102–105, discussion: 106–109.

Schwartz, A. L. (2000). Daily fatigue patterns and effect of exercise in women with breast cancer. *Cancer Practice, 8*(1), 16–24.

Seay, T. M., Blute, M. C., & Zincke, H. (1997). Radical prostatectomy and early adjuvant hormonal therapy for pTxN+ adenocarcinoma of the prostate. *Urology, 50*(6), 835–837.

Selby, P. J., Chapman, J. A. W., Etazadi-Amoli, J., Dalley, D., & Boyd, N. F. (1984). The development of a method for assessing the quality of life of cancer patients. *British Journal of Cancer, 50,* 13–22.

Sellick, S., & Crooks. D. L. (1999). Depression and cancer: An appraisal of the literature for the prevalence, detection, and practice guideline development for psychological interventions. *Psycho-oncology, 8,* 315–333.

Serafini, A. N., Houston, S. J., Resche, I., Quick, D. P., Grund, F. M., Ell, P. J., Bertrand, A., Ahmann, F. R., Orihuela, E., Reid, R. H., Lerski, R. A., Collier, B. D., McKillop, J. H., Purnell, G. L., Pecking, A. P., Thomas, F. D., & Harrison, K. A. (1998). Palliation of pain associated with metastatic bone cancer using samarium-153 lexidronam: A double-blind placebo-controlled clinical trial. *J of Clin Onc, 16,* 1574–1581.

Shelton, P., Weinrich, S., & Reynolds, W. A. Jr. (1999). Barriers to prostate cancer screening in African American men. *Journal of National Black Nurses Association, 10*(2), 14–28.

Shipley, W. U., Zietman, A. L., Hanks, G. E., Coen, J. J., Caplan, R. J., Won, M., Zagars, G. K., & Asbell, S. O. (1994). Treatment related sequelae following external beam radiation for prostate cancer: A review with an update in patients with stage T1 and T2 tumor. *J Urol, 152,* 1799–1805.

Shrader-Bogen, C., Kjellberg, J., McPherson, C., & Murray, C. (1997). Quality of life and treatment outcomes: Prostate carcinoma patients' perspectives after prostatectomy or radiation therapy. *Cancer, 79*(10), 1977–1986.

Sillars, A., & Kalblesch, P. J. (1989). Implicit and explicit decision making styles in couples. In D. Brink & J. Jackard (Eds.), *Dyadic decision making* (pp. 179–201). New York: Springer Verlag.

Sjogren P. (1997). Myoclonic spasms during treatment with high doses of intravenous morphine in renal failure. *Pain, 55*(1), 93–97.

Smathers, S., Wallner, K., Korssjoen, T., Bergsagel, C., Hudson, R. H., Sutlief, S., & Blasko, J. (1999). Radiation safety parameters following prostate brachytherapy. *International Journal of Radiation Oncology, Biology & Physics, 45*(2), 397–399.

Skander, M. P., & Ryan, F. P. (1988). Non-steroidal anti-inflammatory drugs and pain free peptic ulceration in the elderly. *BMJ, 297,* 833–834.

Smeenk F. W., de Witte L. P., Van Haastregt J. C., Schipper R. M., Biezeman H. P., & Crebolder H. F. (1998). Transmural Care of Terminal Cancer Patients. *Nurs Res, 47*(3), 129–136.

Smith, D. B. (1999). Urinary incontinence issues in oncology. *Clinical Journal of Oncology Nursing, 3*(4).

Smith, D. S., Bullock, A. D., Catalona, W. J., & Herschman, J. D. (1996).

Racial differences in a prostate cancer screening study. *Journal of Urology, 156,* 1366–1369.
Smith, P. L., Britt, E. J., Terry, P. B. : Common pulmonary problems, in Barker, L. R., Burton, J. R., Zieve, P. D. (Eds.), *Principles of Ambulatory Medicine* (4th ed., pp. 633–650). Baltimore, MD: Williams & Wilkins.
Smith, R. A., von Eschenbach, A. C., Wender, R., Levin, B., Byers, T., Rothenbrger, D., Brooks, D., Creasman, W., Cohen, C., Runowicz, C., Cokkinides, V., & Eyre, H. (2001). American Cancer Society guidelines for the early detection of cancer: Update of early detection guidelines for prostate, colorectal, and endometrial cancers. *CA: A Cancer Journal for Clinicians, 51*(1), 38–75.
Smith, R. A., Mettlin, C. J., Davis, D. J., & Eyre, H. (2000). American Cancer Society guidelines for the early detection of cancer. *CA: A Cancer Journal for Clinicians, 50*(1), 34–49.
Snyder, G. (2000). Prostate cancer. In B. M. Nevidjon & K. W. Sowers (Eds.), *A nurse's guide to cancer care* (pp. 122–134). Philadelphia: Lippincott.
Sommers, S., & Ramsey, S. (1999). A review of quality-of-life evaluations in prostate cancer. *Pharmacoeconomics, 16*(2), 127–140.
Soucheck, J., Stacks, J. R., Brody, B., Ashton, C. M., Geiser, R. B., Byrne, M. M., Cook, K., Geraci, J. M., & Wray, N. P. (2000). A trial for comparing methods of eliciting treatment preferences for men with advanced prostate cancer: Results from initial visit. *Medical Care, 38,* 1040–1050.
Spiegel, D. (1990). Can psychotherapy prolong cancer survival? *Psychosomatics, 31,* 361–366.
Spiegel, D., Bloom, J., & Yalom, I. (1981). Group support for patients with metastatic cancer. *Archives of General Psychiatry, 38,* 527–533.
Spitz, M. R., Currier, R. D., Fueger, J. J., Babaian, R. J., & Newell, G. R. (1991). Family patterns of prostate cancer: A case-control analysis. *Journal of Urology, 146,* 1305–1307.
Sporkin, E. (1992). Patient and family education. In K. H. Dow, & L. Hilderley (Eds.), *Nursing Care in Radiation Oncology.* Philadelphia: Saunders.
Stanford, J., Feng, Z., Hamilton, A., Gilliland, F., Stephenson, R., Eley, J., Albertsen, P., Harlan, L., & Potosky, A. (20001). Urinary and sexual function after radical prostatectomy for clinically localized prostate cancer: The Prostate Cancer Outcomes Study. *Journal of the American Medical Association, 19, 283*(3), 354–360.
Stedman's Medical Dictionary (1990). (25th ed., p. 733). Baltimore, MD: Williams & Wilkins.
Steele, G. S., Sullivan, M. P., Sleep, D. J., & Yalla, S. V. (2000). Combination

of symptom score, flow rate and prostate volume for predicting bladder outflow obstruction in men with lower urinary tract symptoms. *Journal of Urology, 164(2),* 344–348.

Stein, K. D., Martin, S. C., Hann, D. M., & Jacobsen, P. B. (1998). A multidimensional measure of fatigue for use with cancer patients. *Cancer Practice, 6*(3), 143–152.

Steinberg, G. D., Carter, B., S., Beaty, T. H., Child, B., & Walsh, P. C. (1990). Family history and risk of prostate cancer. *Prostate, 17,* 337–347.

Stempkowski, L. (2000). Hormonal therapy. In J. Held-Warmkessel (Ed.) *Contemporary issues in prostate cancer* (pp. 170–189). Sudbury, MA: Jones and Bartlett Publishers.

Stempkowski, L. (2000). Hormonal therapy. In J. Held-Warmkessel (Ed.), *Contemporary issues in prostate cancer: A nursing perspective* (pp. 170–194). Boston: Jones and Bartlett Publishers.

Stenman, U. H., Leinonen, J., Alfthan, H., Raannikko, S., Tuhkanen, K., & Alfthan, O. (1991). A complex between prostate-specific antigen and a 1-antichumotrypsin is the major form of prostate-specific antigen in serum of patients with prostate cancer: Essay of the comple improves clinical sensitivity for cancer. *Cancer Research, 51,* 222–226.

Stock R. (1995). Locoregional therapies for early stage prostate cancer. *Oncology, 9,* 803–815.

Surveillance, Epidemiology, and End Results (SEER) Program Public-Use CD-ROM (1973-1997), National Cancer Institute, DCCPS, Cancer Surveillance Research Program, Cancer Statistics Branch, released April 2000, based on the August 1999 submission. U. S. Department of Health and Human Services: Healthy people 2010: National health promotion and disease prevention objectives, http://www. health. gov/healthypeople.

Swan, D. K., & Ford, B. (1997). Chemoprevention of cancer: Review of the literature. *Oncology Nursing Forum, 24*(4), 719–727.

Talcott, J. A., Reiker, P, Clark, J. A., Propert, K. J., Weeks, J. C., Beard, C. J., Wishnow, K. I., Kaplan, I., Loughlin, K. R., Richie, J. P, & Kantoff, P. W. (1998). Patient-reported symptoms after primary therapy for early prostate cancer: Results of a prospective cohort study. *Journal of Clinical Oncology, 16,* 275–283.

Tannock, I. F., Osoba, D., Stockler, M. R., Ernst, D. S., Neville, A. J., Moore, M. J., Armitage, G. R., Wilson, J. J., Venner, P. M., Coppin, C. M., & Murphy, K. C. (1996). Chemotherapy with Mitoxantrone plus Prednisone or Prednisone alone for symptomatic hormone-resistant prostate cancer: A Canadian randomized trial with palliative end-points. *J Clin Oncol June 14*(6), 1756–1764.

Terk, M. D., Stock, R. G., & Stone, N. N. (1998). Identification of patients at increased risk for prolonged urinary retention following radioactive seed implantation of the prostate. *Journal of Urology, 160,* 1379–1382.

Teshima, T., Hanks, G. E., Hanlon, A. L., Peter, R. S., & Schultheiss, T. E. (1997). Rectal bleeding after conformal 3D treatment of prostate cancer: Time to occurrence, response to treatment and duration of morbidity. *International Journal of Radiation Oncology Biology & Physics, 39,* 77–83.

Tester, W., & Brouch, M. D. (2000). Treatment decision making. In J. Held-Warmkessel (Ed.), *Contemporary issues in prostate cancer: A nursing perspective* (pp. 81–101). Boston: Jones-Bartlett.

Thompson, I., Feigl, P., & Coltman, C. (1996). Chemoprevention of prostate cancer with Finasteride. In V. T. DeVita, Jr., S. Hellman, & S. A. Rosenberg (Eds.), *Principles and practice of oncology updates, 10*(3), pp. 1–18. Philadelphia: Lippincott-Raven.

Thompson, I. M., Middleton, R. G., Optenberg, S. A., Austenfeld, M. S., Smalley, S. R., Cooner, W. H., Correa, R. J., Miller, H. C., Oesterling, J. E., Resnick, M. I., Wasson, J. H., & Roehrborn, C. G. (1999). Have complication rates decreased after treatment for localized prostate cancer? *The Journal of Urology, 162*(1), 107–112.

Tingen, M. S., Weinrich, S. P., Heyolt, D. D., Boyd, M. D., & Weinrich, M. C. (1998). Perceived benefits: A predictor of participation in prostate cancer screening. *Cancer Nursing, 21,* 349–357.

Tofe, A. J., Francis, M. D., & Harvey W. J. (1975). Correlation of neoplasms with incidence and localization of bone metastases: An analysis of 1355 diphosphonate bone scans. *J Nucl Med, 16,* 986–989.

Tunkel, R. S., & Rampulla, P. (1998). Lymphedema: Current treatments and controversies. In R. K. Portenoy & E. Bruera (Eds.), *Topics in palliative care* (vol. 3, pp. 271–283). New York: Oxford University Press.

Turner, S. L., Adams, K., Bull, C. A., & Berry, M. P. (1999). Sexual dysfunction after radical radiation therapy for prostate cancer: A prospective evaluation. *Urology, 54*(1), 124–129.

Underwood, S. (1991). African-American men: Perceptual determinations of early cancer detection and cancer risk reduction. *Cancer Nursing, 14,* 281–288.

U. S. Preventive Services Task Force. (1996). *Guide to clinical preventive services* (2nd ed.). Baltimore: Williams & Wilkins.

Valanis, B., & Rumpler, C. (1982). Healthy women's perspectives on breast cancer treatment. *Journal of the American Medical Women's Association, 37,* 311–316.

Varnus, H. E. (1999, June). Planning for prostate cancer research. Expanding

References

the scientific framework: The burden of prostate cancer. *National Institute of Health.* Available www. nci. gov/prostateplan3. html.

Vashi, A. R., Wojno, K. J., Henricks, W. England B. A., Vessella, R. L., Lange, P. H., Wright, G. L., Schellhammer, P. F., Weigand, R. A., Dowell, B. L., & Borden, K. K. (1997). Determination of the "reflex range" and appropriate cutpoints for percent free prostate-specific antigen in 413 men referred for prostatic evaluation using the AxSym system. *Urology, 49,* 19–27.

Ventafridda, V., Ripamonti, C., DeConno, Tamburini, M., & Cassileth, B. R. (1990). Symptom prevalence and control during cancer patients' last days of life. *J Palliat Care, 6*(3), 7–11.

Vestal, R. (1997). Aging and pharmacology. *Cancer 80*(7), 1302–1310.

Vetrosky, D., & White, G. L. Jr. (1998). Prostate cancer: Clinical perspectives. *American Association of Occupational Health Nurse Journal, 46,* 434–440.

Villejo, L., & Meyers, C. (1991). Brain function, learning styles, and cancer patient education. *Seminars in Oncology Nursing, 7,* 97–104.

Villeneuve, P. J., Johnson, K. C., Kreiger, N., Maa, Y., & The Canadian Cancer Registries Epidemiology Research Group (1999). Risk factors for prostate cancer: Results from the Canadian National Enhanced Cancer Surveillance System. *Cancer Causes and Control, 10,* 355–367.

Volk, R. J., Cantor, S. B., Spann, S. J., Cass, A. R., Cardenas, M. P, & Warren, M. M. (1997). Preferences of husbands and wives for prostate cancer screening. *Archives of Family Medicine, 6,* 72–76.

Volk, R. J., Cass, A. R., & Spann, S. J. (1999). A randomized controlled trial of shared decision making for prostate cancer screening. *Archives of Family Medicine, 8,* 333–340.

Volker, D. L. (1998). Application of the standards of practice and education. In J. K. Itano & K. N. Taoka (Eds.), *Core curriculum for oncology nursing* (3rd ed., pp. 713–726). Philadelphia: W. B. Saunders.

Von Eschenbach, A., Ho, R., Murphy, G. P., Cunningham, M., & Lins, N. (1997). American cancer society guidelines for the early detection of prostate cancer. *Cancer, 80,* 1805–1807.

Von Roenn, J. H., Cleeland, C. S., Gonin, R., Hatfield, A. K., & Pandya, K. J. (1993). Physician attitudes and practice in cancer pain management: A survey from the Eastern Cooperative Oncology Group. *Ann Intern Med, 119*(2), 121–126.

Waldman, A. R., & Osborne, D. M. (1994). Screening for prostate cancer. *Oncology Nursing Forum, 21,* 1513–1517.

Wallace, M. (2001). *The quality of life of older men receiving the watchful waiting treatment for prostate cancer.* Unpublished doctoral dissertation, New York University.

Wallner, K., Roy, J., Zelefsky, M., Fuks, Z., Harrison, L. (1994). Fluoroscopic visualization of the prostatic urethra to guide transperineal prostate implantation. *International Journal of Radiation Oncology Biology Physics, 29,* 863–867.

Wallner, K., Lee, H., Wasserman, S., Dattol, M. (1997). Low risk of urinary incontinence following prostate brachytherapy in patients with a prior transurethral prostate resection. *International Journal of Radiation Oncology Biology and Physics, 37,* 565–569.

Walsh, P. C. (1998). Anatomic radical retropubic prostatectomy. In P. C. Walsh, A. B. Retik, E. D. Jr., Vaughan, & A. J. Wein (Eds.), *Campbells' urology* (7th ed., pp. 2565–2587). Philadelphia, PA: Saunders.

Walsh, P. C., & Donker, P. J. (1982). Impotence following radical prostatectomy: Insight into etiology and prevention. *Journal of Urology, 128,* 492–497.

Walsh, P. C., Marsche, P., Ricker, D., & Burnett, A. L. (2000). Patient reported urinary continence and sexual functioning after anatomic radical prostatectomy. *Urology, 55,* 58–61.

Walsh, P. C., & Partin, A. W. (1997). Family history facilities the early diagnosis of prostate carcinoma. *Cancer, 80,* 1871–1874.

Walsh, P. C., Partin, A. W., & Epstein, J. I. (1994). Cancer control and quality of life following anatomical radical retropubic prostatectomy: Results at 10 years. *Journal of Urology, 152,* 1831–1836.

Walsh, P. C., & Worthington, J. F. (1995). *The prostate: A guide for men and the women that love them.* Baltimore, MD: The Johns Hopkins University Press.

Walther, P. J. (1999). Interstitial brachytherapy for prostate cancer—Just an expensive variant of "watchful waiting"? *Current Opinion in Urology, 9,* 201–204.

Ward, S. E., Goldberg, N., Miller-McCauley, V., Mueller, C., Nolan, A., Pawlik-Plank, D., Robbins, A., Stormoen, D., & Weissman, D. E. (1993). Patient-related barriers to management of cancer pain. *Pain, 52*(3), 319–324.

Ward, S., Heidrich, S., & Wolberg, W. (1989). Factors women take into account when deciding on type of surgery for breast cancer. *Cancer Nusing, 12,* 344–351.

Ware, J. (1984). Conceptualizing disease impact and treatment outcomes. *Cancer, 10*(53), 2317–2326.

Ware, J. E., & Sherbourne, C. D. (1992). The MOS 36-item short-form health survey (SF-36): Conceptual framework and item selection. *Medical Care, 30,* 473.

Waxman, E. S. (1993). Sexual dysfunction following treatment for prostate cancer: Nursing assessment and interventions. *Oncology Nursing Forum, 20*(10), 1567–1571.

Weber, B. A., Roberts, B. L., & McDougall, G. J. Jr. (2000). Exploring the efficacy of support groups for men with prostate cancer. *Geriatric Nursing, 21*(5), 250–253.

Wei, J. T., Dunn, R. L., Marcovich, R., Montie, J. E., & Sanda, M. G. (2000). Prospective assessment of patient reported urinary continence after radical prostatectomy. *Journal of Urology, 164*(3 Pt 1), 744–748.

Weinrich, S. P., Reynolds, W. A., Tingen, M. S., & Starr, C. R. (2000). Barriers to prostate cancer screening. *Cancer Nursing, 23*(2), 117–122.

Weinrich, S. P., Weinrich, M. C., Boyd, M. D., & Atkinson, C. (1998). The impact of prostate cancer knowledge on cancer screening. *Oncology Nursing Forum, 25*(3), 527–534.

Weissman, D. E., Dahl, J. L., & Beasley, J. W. (1993). The cancer pain role model program of the Wisconsin cancer pain initiative. *J Pain Symptom Manage, 8*, 29–35.

Weldon, V. E., Tavel, F. R., & Newirth, H. (1997). Continence, potency and morbidity after radical perineal prostatectomy. *Journal of Urology, 158*(4), 1470–1475.

Whitman-Obert, H. H. (1996). Patient information handouts: Taking care of yourself-A self-help guide for patients with cancer. *Oncology Nursing Forum, 23*(9), 1443–1445.

Whittemore, A. S., Wu, A. H., Kolonel, L. N., John, E. M., Gallagher, R. P., Howe, G. R., West, D. W., The, C. Z., & Stamey, T. (1995). Family history and prostate cancer risk in Black, White, and Asian men in the United States and Canada. *American Journal of Epidemiology, 141*, 732–740.

Wilson, K. G., Chochinov, H. M., de Faye, B. J., & Breitbart. W. (2000). Diagnosis and management of depression in palliative care. In H. M. Chochinovrt (Ed.), *Handbook of psychiatry in palliative medicine* (pp. 25–49). New York: Oxford University Press.

Winningham, M. L., Nail, L. M., Burke, M. B., Brophy, L., Cimprich, B., Jones, L. S., Pickard-Holley, S., Rhodes, V., St. Pierre, B., Beck, S., Glass, E. C., Mock, V. L., Mooney, K. H., & Piper, B. (1994). Fatigue and the cancer experience: The state of the knowledge. *Oncology Nursing Forum, 21*(1), 23–36.

Wolfe, C. M. (1960). An investigation of familial aspects of carcinoma of the prostate. *Cancer, 13*, 739–744.

Wolfe, M. E., Lichtenstein, D. R., & Sing, G. (1999). Gastrointestinal toxicity of nonsteroidal antiinflammatory drugs. *New Eng J Med, 340*(24), 1888–1899.

Wong, W. S, Chinn, D. O, Chinn, M., & Tom W. L. (1997). Cryosurgery as a treatment for prostate cancer: Results and complications. *Cancer, 79*, 963–974.

Wood, C. K., & Lockhart, J. S. (2000). Prostate cancer. *American Journal of Nursing, 200*(Suppl 4), 47–51.
World Health Organization. (1999). *Cancer pain relief* (2nd ed.). (WHO Technical Report Series, No. 804). Geneva, Switzerland.
World Health Organization. (1976). Education and trends in human sexuality: The training of health care professionals (Technical Report Series No. 572). Geneva, Switzerland: Author.
World Health Organization. (1958). *The first ten years of the World Health Organization.* Geneva: World Health Organization.
Wortman, C. (1984). Social support and the cancer patient: Conceptual and methodologic issues. *Cancer(supp), 53,* 2339–2360.
Wu, A., Cagney, K., & St. John, P. (1997). Health status assessment. Completing the clinical database. *Journal of General Internal Medicine, 12*(4), 203–208.
Yan, Y., Carvalhal, G. F., Catalona, W. J., & Young, J. D. (2000). Primary treatment choices for men with clinically localized prostate carcinoma detected by screening. *Cancer, 88,* 1122–1130.
Yarbro, C. H., & Ferrans, C. E. (1998). Quality of life of patients with prostate cancer treated with surgery or radiation therapy. *Oncology Nursing Forum, 25,* 685–693.
Yellen, S. B., & Cella, D. F. (1995). Someone to live for: Social well-being, parenthood status, and decision-making in oncology. *Journal of Clinical Oncology, 13,* 1255–1264.
Yellen, S. B., Cella, D. F., Webster, K., Blendowski, C., & Kaplan, E. (1997). Measuring fatigue and other anemia-related symptoms with the Functional Assessment of Cancer Therapy (FACT) measurement system. *Journal of Pain & Symptom Management, 13*(2), 63–74.
Yeoh, E. K., Russo, A., Botten, R., Fraser, R., Roos, D., Penniment, M., Borg, M., & Sun, W. M. (1998). Acute effects of therapeutic irradiation for prostatic carcinoma on anorectal function. *Gut, 43*(1), 123–127.
Yoshizawa, K., Willet, W., Morris, S. J., Stampfer, M. J., Spiegelman, D., Rimm, E., & Giovannucci, E. (1998). Study of prediagnostic selenium level in toenails and the risk of advanced prostate cancer. *Journal of the National Cancer Institute, 90,* 1219–1224.
Zampini, K., & Ostroff, J. S. (1993). The post-treatment resource program: Portrait of a program for cancer survivors. *Psyco-oncology, 2,* 1–9.
Zelefsky, M. J., Ginor, R. X., & Leibel, S. A. (1999). Efficacy of selective alpha-1 blocker therapy in the treatment of acute urinary symptoms during radiotherapy for localized prostate cancer. *International Journal of Radiation Oncology Biology & Physics, 45*(3), 567–570.
Ziada, A., Rosenblum, M., & Crawford, D. (2000). Hormonal Therapy:

Neoadjuvant, adjuvant, and intermittent. In E. A. Klein (Ed.), *Management of Prostate Cancer* (pp. 265–288). Totowa, NJ: Humana Press.

Zippe, C. D., Jhaveri, F. M., Klein, E. A., Kedia, S., Pasqualotto, F. F., Kedia, A., Agarwal, A., Montague, D. K., Lakin, M. M. (2000). Role of Viagra after radical prostatectomy. *Urology,* 55(2), 241–245, 309.

Zlotta, A. R., & Schulman, C. C. (1998). Etiology and diagnosis of prostate cancer: What's new? *European Urology, 33,* 351–358.

Index

Acetaminophen, 171
ACS. See American Cancer Society
Actis ring, 86
Advocates, role of nurses as, 29
Age, prostate cancer and, 4, 16–17
   decision-making preferences and, 50–51
   serum prostate-specific antigen, 37
Alcohol consumption, 25, 171
Alkaline phosphatase, elevation of, 44
Alpha reductase, 26
Alprazolam, 167
Alprostadil, 149
American Cancer Society, 142
Analgesia, 163
Anatomy, prostate cancer, 6–7
Androgen, 111
   blockade, combined, 112
   deprivation therapy, 23
Anemia, 165–166
   colony-stimulating factor, 100
   fatigue and, 100
   lymphedema, 165–166
Antiandrogen agents, 114–115
Anticholinergics, 171
Anticonvulsants agents, 171
Antidepressants, 171
Antiemetics, 171
Antihistamines, 171
Antihypertensives, 171
Antineoplastics, 171
Antiparkinson agents, 171
Antispasmodics, 171
   radical prostatectomy, 81

Anxiety, 167–168
   fatigue and, 100
   in men with prostate cancer, 152
AOSW. See Association of Oncology Social Workers
Assessment of patient, 33–45
   digital rectal examination, 37
   prostate-specific antigen, combined use of, 37–38
   prostate-specific antigen test, 34–37
   symptom pattern, 33–34
   transrectal ultrasonography, 38–40
Association of Oncology Social Workers, 143
Australia, incidence of prostate cancer in, 5

Band use, for erectile dysfunction, radical prostatectomy, 86
Benign prostatic hyperplasia, 23
Benzodiazepines, 167
Beta-carotene, 21
BFI. See Brief Fatigue Inventory
Biases, treatment-related, 57–58
Bisphosphonates, 161–163
Bladder spasms, radical prostatectomy associated with, 84
Blockade, sympathetic, for pain, 163–164
Bone pain
   radiation therapy for, 162
   Samarium-153, 143
   Strontium-89, 143
Bone-seeking radioisotopes, 163

Bowel dysfunction, treatment-related, 51, 53
BPH. *See* Benign prostatic hyperplasia
Brachytherapy, 101, 108
   postoperative care of, 93–94
   rectal symptoms associated with, 107
   safety precautions, 94–95
   seed implantation, 91–96
   urinary symptoms, 101
Breast tenderness, as side effect of hormone therapy, 124
Brief Fatigue Inventory, 99

CAB. *See* Combined androgen blockade
Cadmium, environmental exposure to, 22
Calcium, elevation of, 44
Canada, incidence of prostate cancer in, 5
Cancer Care, Inc., 142
Cancer Rehabilitation Evaluation Survey Short Form, 65, 70
Cancer-specific quality of life, 65–67
   instruments, 68
Cancer Survivor Toolbox, 143
Caregiver issues, 172
CARES. *See* Cancer Rehabilitation Evaluation Survey Short Form
Catheter care, radical prostatectomy, 80
Celiac plexus block, for pain, 163–164
Cellular classification, prostate cancer, 9–12
Cervicothoracic ganglion block, for pain, 163–164
Chemoprevention, 25–28
Chemotherapy, 119–121, 124
China, incidence of prostate cancer in, 5
Chinese population, incidence of prostate cancer in, 6
Cigarette smoking, 24
Clonazepam, 167
Coban, 86
Codeine, 158–159, 160
Cognitive-behavioral interventions, 164
   guided imagery, 164
   music therapy, 164
   relaxation, 164

Colony-stimulating factor, for anemia, 100
Combined androgen blockade, 112
Complementary therapies, for pain, 164
Complete androgen blockade, 115–116
Computed tomography, 44
Condition-specific quality of life, 67–70
Cordotomy, 163–164
Corticosteroids, 171
Costa Rica, incidence of prostate cancer in, 5

Decision-making process, 46–61
Deep venous thrombosis, radical prostatectomy, 82
Delirium, 169–171
   drugs causing, 171
Demerol, 158–160
Denmark, incidence of prostate cancer in, 5
Depression, 168–169
   fatigue and, 100
DES. *See* Diethylstilbestrol
Deta-4-androstenedione, 111
DFMO. *See* Difuromethylornithine
DHEA. *See* Dihydroepiandrosterone
Diabetic agents, 171
Diagnosis, 33–45
   alkaline phosphatase, elevation of, 44
   calcium, elevation of, 44
   computed tomography, 44
   diagnostic testing, 43–44
   grading, 44–45
   radionuclide bone scan, 44
   staging, 44–45
   transrectal biopsy, 43
Diet, 20–21
Diethylstilbestrol, 113
Difuromethylornithine, 28
Digital rectal examination, 38
Dihydroepiandrosterone, 111
Dihydrotestosterone, 26
Dioxyribonucleic acid, zinc and, 22
Discharge planning, radical prostatectomy, 82–84
   catheter care, 83–84
   erectile function, 84

Index

pain management, postoperative, 84
postoperative complications, 82–83
urinary continence, 83–84
Ditropan, 81
DNA. *See* Dioxyribonucleic acid
Dysuria, 35

Economic issues, watchful waiting, 138–139
Economic issues, 28–29, 138–139
  digital rectal examination, prostate-specific antigen measurement, cost-effectiveness, 29
Education, patient, 140–152
  American Cancer Society, 142
  anxiety, in men with prostate cancer, 152
  Association of Oncology Social Workers, 143
  bone pain
    Samarium-153, 143
    Strontium-89, 143
  Cancer Care, Inc., 142
  Cancer Survivor Toolbox, 143
  chemotherapy, 124
  family education, 141–143
  Health Related Quality of Life, 144
  helplessness, in men with prostate cancer, 152
  importance of, 30
  incontinence assessment, questions, 145
  intraurethral alprostadil, 149
  isolation, in men with prostate cancer, 152
  Man to Man, support groups, 151
  National Cancer Institute, 142
  National Coalition of Cancer Survivors, 142, 143
  Oncology Nursing Society, 143
  oral erectogenic agents, 148–149
  psychosexual therapy, 149
  psychosocial issues, 150–152
  sexual dysfunction, 147–150
  support groups, 151
  University of California at Los Angeles–Prostate Cancer Inventory, 144
  urinary incontinence, 143–146
  vacuum constriction device, 149
  Viagra, 148–149
  worthlessness, sense of, in men with prostate cancer, 152
Electrolyte management, radical prostatectomy, 80–81
End of life care, 153–172
  adjuvants, 159–161
  anemia, 165–166
    lymphedema, 165–166
  anxiety, 167–168
  assessment, 156
  benzodiazepines, 167
  bisphosphonates, 161–163
  care plan, 155
  delirium, 169–171
    drugs causing, 171
  depression, 168–169
  family/caregiver issues, 172
  fatigue, 164–165
  hospice care, 172
  hydronephrosis, 166
  McGill Pain Questionnaire, 157
  opioids, 158–160
  pain, 154–164
    assessment instruments, 157
    barriers to management, 156–158
    complementary therapies, 164
    nonpharmacological approaches, 164
    surgical approaches, 163–164
  pharmacology, 161
  radioisotopes, 161–163
  radiotherapy, 161–163
England, incidence of prostate cancer in, 5
Environmental exposure, 22–23
EORTC-C-33. *See* European Organization for Research and Treatment of Cancer-Quality of Life Questionnaire-C-33
Epidemiology, 1–3
  incidence, 2
  prevalence, 2–3

Epogen, 100
Erectile dysfunction, 86, 122, 147–150
  after radical prostatectomy, 86–87
  radiation, 108
Erectogenic agents, oral, 148–149
Estradiol level, 20
Ethical issues, 28–29
  with watchful waiting, 138–139
Ethnicity, 3–6, 17–18
  serum prostate-specific antigen, 37
European Organization for Research and Treatment of Cancer-Quality of Life Questionnaire-C-33, 65
External beam radiation, 90–91, 101, 105–106

FACT. *See* Functional Assessment of Cancer Therapy
FACT-F. *See* Functional Assessment of Cancer Therapy–Fatigue Subscale
FACT-G. *See* Functional Assessment of Cancer Therapy–General Form
Family education, 141–143
Family history, 18–19
Family issues, end of life care, 172
Family support, watchful waiting and, 135–136
Fat consumption, 20
Fatigue, 164–165
  management, 99–101
  with radiation, 96–101
  as side effect of hormone therapy, 123
Fentanyl patch, 158–160
Filipino population, incidence of prostate cancer in, 6
Financial burden, 28
Finasteride, 26
Finland, incidence of prostate cancer in, 5
France, incidence of prostate cancer in, 5
Frequency, 35
Functional Assessment of Cancer Therapy, 65
Functional Assessment of Cancer Therapy–Fatigue Subscale, 99

Functional Assessment of Cancer Therapy–General Form, 70
Funding issues, watchful waiting, 138–139

Germany, incidence of prostate cancer in, 5
Global quality of life, 64–65
  instruments, 66
Grading, prostate cancer, 44–45
Guided imagery, 164
Gynecomastia, as side effect of hormone therapy, 124

H^2 receptor antagonists, 171
Hawaiian population, incidence of prostate cancer in, 6
Health Related Quality of Life, 144
Height, prostate cancer and, 25
Helplessness, in men with prostate cancer, 152
Hematuria, 35
Hemorrhoidal irritation, with radiation, 106
Heredity, 19–20
High dose rate brachytherapy, 108. *See also* Brachytherapy
High-fat diet, 20
High-fiber diet, 20
Historical perspective, 15–16
Hong Kong, incidence of prostate cancer in, 5
Hormone refractory prostate cancer, 117–119
Hormone therapy, 23–24, 110–125
  androgen blockade
    combined, 112
    complete, 115–116
  androgens, 111
  antiandrogen agent, 114
  antiandrogen medications, 114–115
  breast tenderness, as side effect of hormone therapy, 124
  changing urinary symptoms, 117
  chemotherapy, 119–121
  deta-4-androstenedione, 111
  diethylstilbestrol, 113

Index

dihydroepiandrosterone, 111
  effect on prostate tissue growth, 111
  fatigue, as side effect of hormone therapy, 123
  gynecomastia, as side effect of hormone therapy, 124
  hormone refractory prostate cancer, 117–119
  hot flashes, as side effect of hormone therapy, 122
  impotence, as side effect of hormone therapy, 123
  intermittent hormone therapy, 116–117
  libido, decreased, 123
  Lupron, 114
  luteinizing hormone, 112
  luteinizing hormone releasing hormone, 112
  luteinizing hormone releasing hormone agonist, 113, 116
  luteinizing hormone releasing hormone stimulation, 113
  Man to Man, support groups, 124
  Megace, 115
  nursing implications, 121–124
  osteoporosis, as side effect of hormone therapy, 123
  pain, 117
  patient education, chemotherapy, 124
  prostate cancer support groups, 124
  red flag symptoms, 117
  sexual functioning, 122
  side effects, chemotherapy, 124
  side effects of, 122
  steroidal antiandrogen medications, 115
  types of, 113–114
  Us Too International, 124
  Zoladex, 114
Hospice care, 172
Hot flashes, as side effect of hormone therapy, 122
HRQOL. *See* Health Related Quality of Life
Human papilloma virus, 24
Hydromorphone, 158–160
Hydronephrosis, 166

IGF-1. *See* Insulin-like growth factor
Impotence
  as side effect of treatment, 51–52, 123
IMRT. *See* Intense modulated radiation therapy
Incontinence. *See* Urinary incontinence
India, incidence of prostate cancer in, 5
Insulin-like growth factor, 20
Intense modulated radiation therapy, 108
Intermittent hormone therapy, 116–117
International incidence rates, 5
Intracorporeal injection therapy, radical prostatectomy, 86
Intrapleural opioids, 163
Intraventricular analgesia, 163
Ireland, incidence of prostate cancer in, 5
Isolation, in men with prostate cancer, 152
Israel, incidence of prostate cancer in, 5
Italy, incidence of prostate cancer in, 5

Japan, incidence of prostate cancer in, 5

Korean population, incidence of prostate cancer in, 6

Laparoscopic prostatectomy, 78–79
LHRH. *See* Luteinizing hormone releasing hormone
Libido, decreased, 123
Lithium, 171
Lorazepam, 167
Los Angeles, incidence of prostate cancer in, 5
Lupron, 114
Luteinizing hormone, 112
Luteinizing hormone releasing hormone, 112
  agonist, 113, 116
  stimulation, 113
Lycopenes, protective effects of, 21
Lymphedema, 165–166

Managed care plans, lack of financial support by, 31
Man to Man, support groups, 124, 151
McGill Pain Questionnaire, 157
Medical considerations, treatment decisions and, 48
Medical models, 47
Medicare, lack of financial support by, 31
Megace, 115
Methadone, 158–160
MFSI. *See* Multidimensional Fatigue Symptom Inventory
Morphine, 158–160
  with radical prostatectomy, 81
Mortality, 11–12
  with watchful waiting, 130–133
MPQ. *See* McGill Pain Questionnaire
MQOLS-CA. *See* Multidimensional Quality of Life Scale-Cancer
Multidimensional Fatigue Symptom Inventory, 99
Multidimensional Quality of Life Scale-Cancer, 65
Multiple sexual partners, 24
Music therapy, 164

National Cancer Institute, 142
National Coalition of Cancer Survivors, 142, 143
National Institutes of Health, prostate cancer research funding by, 29
Native American population, incidence of prostate cancer in, 6
NCI. *See* National Cancer Institute
Netherlands, incidence of prostate cancer in, 5
Neurolytic procedures, for pain, 163–164
New Zealand, incidence of prostate cancer in, 5
Nocturia, 35
Nonsteroidal anti-inflammatory agents, 171
Norway, incidence of prostate cancer in, 5
NRS. *See* Numeric Rating Scale
Numeric Rating Scale, 157

Obesity, 25
Occupational exposure, 22–23
Oncology Nursing Society, 143
ONS. *See* Oncology Nursing Society
Opioids, 158–160, 171
  intrapleural, 163
Oral erectogenic agents, 148–149
Osteoporosis, as side effect of hormone therapy, 123
Oxybutynin chloride, 81
Oxycodone, 158–160

Pain, 117, 154–164
  assessment instruments, 157
  barriers to management, 156–158
  bone
    radiation therapy for, 162
    Samarium-153, 143
    Strontium-89, 143
  complementary therapies, 164
  nonpharmacological approaches, 164
  radical prostatectomy, 81
  surgical approaches, 163–164
Pathophysiology, prostate cancer, 6–7
Pathway ablation procedure, for pain, 163–164
Patient advocates, role of nurses as, 29
Patient education, 140–152
  American Cancer Society, 142
  anxiety, in men with prostate cancer, 152
  Association of Oncology Social Workers, 143
  bone pain
    Samarium-153, 143
    Strontium-89, 143
  Cancer Care, Inc., 142
  Cancer Survivor Toolbox, 143
  chemotherapy, 124
  family education, 141–143
  Health Related Quality of Life, 144
  helplessness, in men with prostate cancer, 152
  incontinence assessment, questions, 145
  intraurethral alprostadil, 149

isolation, in men with prostate cancer, 152
Man to Man, support groups, 151
National Cancer Institute, 142
National Coalition of Cancer Survivors, 142, 143
Oncology Nursing Society, 143
oral erectogenic agents, 148–149
psychosexual therapy, 149
psychosocial issues, 150–152
sexual dysfunction, 147–150
support groups, 151
University of California at Los Angeles–Prostate Cancer Inventory, 144
urinary incontinence, 143–146
vacuum constriction device, 149
Viagra, 148–149
worthlessness, sense of, in men with prostate cancer, 152
Patient preferences, in decision making, 48–50
PCPT. *See* Prostate Cancer Prevention Trial
Penile prostheses, with radical prostatectomy, 86, 87
Perineal prostatectomy, 78–79
Physical activity, 23
Physiology, prostate cancer, 6–7
Piper Fatigue Scale, 99
Poland, incidence of prostate cancer in, 5
Polypharmacy, 161
Prevention of prostate cancer, 14–32
Pro-Banthine, 81
Procrit, 100
Proctitis, with radiation, 105
Propantheline bromide, 81
Propoxyphene, 158–160
Prostate cancer
  assessment, 33–45
  decision-making process, 46–61
  diagnosis, 33–45
  early detection of, 39
  end of life care, 153–172
  hormone therapy, 110–125
  overview, 1–13

patient education, 140–152
prevention, 14–32
prostate specific antigen, 110–125
quality of life with, 62–76
radiation treatment, nursing care for, 89–109
radical prostatectomy, nursing care for, 77–88
risk factors, 14–32
screening, 33–45
support groups, 124
treatment choices, 46–61
watchful waiting, 126–139
Prostate Cancer Prevention Trial, 26
Prostate cancer-specific quality of life instruments, 69
Prostatectomy
  anatomic, radical retropubic prostatectomy, 77
  antispasmodics, 81
  associated with bladder spasms, 84
  band use for erectile dysfunction, 86
  catheter care, 80
  complication prevention, 81
  complications, long-term, 84–88
    erectile dysfunction, 86–87
    prostate-specific antigen, rising, 87–88
    urinary incontinence, 85–86
  deep venous thrombosis, 82
  discharge planning, 82–84
    catheter care, 83–84
    erectile function, 84
    pain management, postoperative, 84
    postoperative complications, 82–83
    urinary continence, 83–84
  fluids, electrolyte management, 80–81
  hospitalization, nursing care during, 79–81
  intracorporeal injection therapy, 86
  laparoscopic, 78–79
  laparoscopic prostatectomy, 78–79
  morphine, 81
  nursing care for, 77–88
  pain management, 81
  penile prostheses, 86, 87
  perineal, 78–79

Prostatectomy *(continued)*
  perineal prostatectomy, 78–79
  retropubic, radical, radical
    prostatectomy, 77
  treatment options, 77–79
  vacuum erection device, 86
  wound care, 80
Prostate specific antigen, 110–125
Prostatic intraepithelial neoplasia, 23
PSA. *See* Prostate-specific antigen
Psychosexual therapy, 149
Psychosocial existential well-being,
  quality of life and, 65
Psychosocial issues, 150–152
Pulmonary embolism, 82

QLI. *See* Quality of Life Index
Quality of life, 10, 62–76
  Cancer Rehabilitation Evaluation
    Survey, Short Form, 65, 70
  cancer-specific quality of life,
    65–68
  condition-specific quality of life,
    67–70
  European Organization for
    Research and Treatment of
    Cancer-Quality of Life
    Questionnaire-C-33, 65
  existential well-being, 65
  Functional Assessment of Cancer
    Therapy, 65
  Functional Assessment of Cancer
    Therapy–General Form, 70
  global quality of life, 64–65
    instruments, 66
  literature summary, 70–76
  measurement issues, 64
  Multidimensional Quality of Life
    Scale-Cancer, 65
  physical functional well-being, 65
  prostate cancer-specific quality of life
    instruments, 69
  psychosocial existential well-being, 65
  Quality of Life Index, 65
  SF-36, 65
  symptom distress, 65
  tools to assess, 31

UCLA Prostate Cancer Index, 70
University of California at
  Los Angeles-Prostate
  Cancer Index, 67
worry, 65

Race, 3–5, 17–18
  distibution, prostate cancer, 6
  serum prostate-specific antigen, 37
Radiation
  anemia, fatigue and, 100
  bone lesion, pain, 162
  brachytherapy, 108
    postoperative care of, 93–94
    rectal symptoms associated with,
      107
    safety precautions, 94–95
    seed implantation, 91–96
    urinary symptoms, 101
  Brief Fatigue Inventory, 99
  colony-stimulating factor, for anemia,
    100
  external beam radiation, 90–91
  fatigue, 96–101
    management, 99–101
  Functional Assessment of Cancer
    Therapy–Fatigue Subscale, 99
  hemorrhoidal irritation, 106
  high dose rate brachytherapy, 108
  intense modulated radiation therapy,
    108
  multidimensional Fatigue Symptom
    Inventory, 99
  nursing care for, 89–109
  Piper Fatigue Scale, 99
  proctitis, 105
  radiosurgery, stereotactic, 108
  rectal symptoms, 105–108
    assessment, 107–108
    external beam radiation, 105–106
    seed implantation/brachytherapy,
      91–96
  sexual dysfunction, 108
  side effects of, 95–98
  sleeping aids, 100
  stereotactic radiosurgery, 108
  treatment options, 89–90

Index

urinary symptoms, 101–105
  assessment, 103–105
  brachytherapy, 101
  external beam radiation, 101
Radical prostatectomy
  anatomic, radical retropubic prostatectomy, 77
  antispasmodics, 81
  associated with bladder spasms, 84
  band use for erectile dysfunction, 86
  catheter care, 80
  complications, 84–88
    erectile dysfunction, 86–87
    prevention of, 81
    prostate-specific antigen, rising, 87–88
    urinary incontinence, 85–86
  deep venous thrombosis, 82
  discharge planning, 82–84
    catheter care, 83–84
    erectile function, 84
    pain management, postoperative, 84
    postoperative complications, 82–83
    urinary continence, 83–84
  fluids, electrolyte management, 80–81
  hospitalization, nursing care during, 79–81
  intracorporeal injection therapy, 86
  laparoscopic prostatectomy, 78–79
  morphine, 81
  nursing care for, 77–88
  pain management, 81
  penile prostheses, 86, 87
  perineal prostatectomy, 78–79
  treatment options, 77–79
  vacuum erection device, 86
  wound care, 80
Radical retropubic prostatectomy, radical prostatectomy, 77
Radioisotopes, 161–163
Radionuclide bone scan, 44
Radiosurgery, stereotactic, 108
Relaxation, 164
Retinoids, 28
Retropubic prostatectomy, radical, radical prostatectomy, 77
Rhizotomy, 163–164

Ribonucleic acid repair, zinc and, 22
Risk factors, for prostate cancer, 14–32
RNA. See Ribonucleic acid repair

Salicylates, 171
Samarium-153, 143
Saw palmetto, 28
Scotland, incidence of prostate cancer in, 5
Screening, for prostate cancer, 10, 33–45
  barriers, 41–42
  for elderly, asymptomatic men, 29
  facilitators, 41–43
  individualized approach for, 42–43
Sedatives, 171
Seed implantation, brachytherapy, 91–96
Selenium, 26, 27
Serenoa repens, 28
Sexual dysfunction, 122, 147–150
  radiation, 108
Side effects
  of chemotherapy, 124
  of radiation, 95–98
  of treatment, 51–52, 56–57
Sildenafil, 148–149
Singapore, incidence of prostate cancer in, 5
Sleep disturbances, fatigue and, 100
Sleeping aids, 100
Smoking, 24
Spain, incidence of prostate cancer in, 5
Spinal analgesia, 163
Staging, 7–8, 44–45
Stereotactic radiosurgery, 108
Steroidal antiandrogen medications, 115
  Cyproterone acetate, 115
Strontium-89, 143
Support groups, 151
Sweden, incidence of prostate cancer in, 5
Switzerland, incidence of prostate cancer in, 5
Sympathetic blockade, for pain, 163–164

Testosterone, 20, 23
Transrectal biopsy, 43
Treatment options, 11, 46–61

University of California at Los Angeles-Prostate Cancer Index, 67, 70, 144
Urinary incontinence, 143–146
  after radical prostatectomy, 85–86
  assessment questions, 145
  as side effect of treatment, 51–61
Us Too International, 124

Vacuum device, penile, 86, 149
VAS. *See* Visual Analogue Scales
Vasectomy, 24
Vegetarian diet, 20
Venereal disease, 24
Viagra, 148–149
Visual Analogue Scales, 157
Vitamin D synthesis, cadmium and, 22
Vitamin E, 26

Wales, incidence of prostate cancer in, 5
Wallace Prostate Cancer Symptom Inventory, 134
Watchful waiting, 126–139
  assessment, 132–133
  characteristics of patients receiving, 128–130
  clinical nursing management, 132
  economic issues, 138–139
  family support, 135–136
  funding issues, 138–139
  literature review, 127
  management, 133–138
  mortality associated with, 130–133
  risks, benefits of, 135
  symptom management, 136–138
  uncertainty, 133–135
    defined, 133
Wallace Prostate Cancer Symptom Inventory, 134
Worry, quality of life and, 65
Worthlessness, sense of, in men with prostate cancer, 152
Wound care, radical prostatectomy, 80

Yugoslavia, incidence of prostate cancer in, 5

Zinc, DNA, RNA repair, 22
Zoladex, 114

The Encyclopedia of Elder Care

The Comprehensive Resource on Geriatric and Social Care

Mathy D. Mezey, RN, EdD, FAAN, Editor-in-Chief
Barbara J. Berkman, DSW, **Christopher M. Callahan,** MD,
Terry T. Fulmer, PhD, RN, FAAN, **Ethel L. Mitty,** EdD, RN,
Gregory J. Paveza, MSW, PhD, **Eugenia L. Siegler,** MD, FACP,
Neville E. Strumpf, PhD, RN, FAAN, Associate Editors
Melissa M. Bottrell, MPH, PhDc, Managing Editor

"THE ENCYCLOPEDIA OF ELDER CARE is an authoritative, comprehensive overview of the best clinical research and practice in contemporary gerontology and geriatrics. Editor Mathy D. Mezey, a distinguished pioneer in elder care, has been joined by many of the nation's most notable scholars and experienced clinicians in producing this timely, readable volume for an aging society."
—**George L. Maddox,** PhD

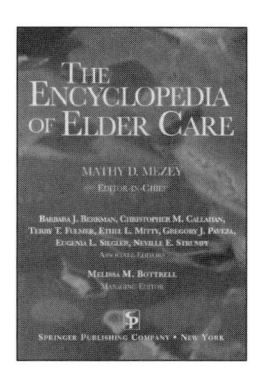

"THE ENCYCLOPEDIA OF ELDER CARE provides a valuable and far-ranging resource for professionals across the whole range of disciplines."
—**Bruce C. Vladeck,** PhD

Caring for elderly individuals requires a command of current information from multiple disciplines. Now, for the first time, this information has been gathered in a single source. Written by experts, this state-of-the-art resource features nearly 300 articles providing practical information on: home care; nursing home care; rehabilitation; case management; social services; assisted living; palliative care; and more. Each article concludes with references to pertinent Web Sites. Easy to read and extensively cross-referenced, the ***Encyclopedia*** is an indispensable tool for all in the caring professions.

2000   824pp   0-8261-1368-0   hardcover

Springer Publishing Company
Palliative Care Nursing
Quality Care to the End of Life
Marianne LaPorte Matzo, PhD, RN, GNP, CS
Deborah Witt Sherman, PhD, RN, ANP, CS, Editors

"This text will be recognized as a foundation for nursing education. The authors ... are recognized leaders in palliative nursing education....The text is a comprehensive approach spanning the traditional to complementary treatments."
—**Betty R. Ferrell,** RN, PhD, FAAN, from the Foreword

This book provides essential information on the best practices for quality care at the end of life. It is organized around the 15 competencies in palliative care developed by the American Association of Colleges of Nursing. The book combines holistic, humanistic caring with aggressive management of pain and symptoms. Comprehensive clinical content is combined with curriculum guidelines for educators. This book is for students and educators at all levels of nursing education, and for practicing nurses working with the terminally ill.

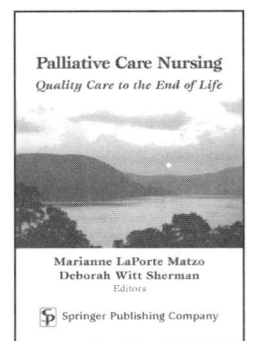

Contents:
Part I. Holistic Aspects of Palliative Care
- Spiritually and Culturally Competent Palliative Care, *D.W. Sherman*
- Holistic Integrative Therapies in Palliative Care, *C. Mariano*

Part II. Social Aspects of Palliative Care
Death and Society, *M. Bookbinder & M. Kiss*
- The Nurse's Roles in Interdisciplinary and Palliative Care, *L.M. Krammer, et al.*
- Ethical Aspects of Palliative Care, *J.K. Schwarz*
- Legal Aspects of Palliative Care, *G.C. Ramsey*

Part III. Psychological Aspects of Dying
- Communicating With Seriously Ill and Dying Patients, Their Families, and Their Health Care Providers, *K.O. Perrin*
- Caring for Families: The Other Patient in Palliative Care, *S.K. Goetschius*
- Loss, Suffering, Bereavement, and Grief, *M.L. Potter*

Part IV. Physical Aspects of Palliative Care
- Symptom Management in Palliative Care, *M.K. Kazanowski*
- Pain Assessment and Management in Palliative Care, *N. Coyle and M. Layman-Goldstein*
- Peri-Death Nursing Care, *M.L. Matzo*

2001   572pp   0-8261-1384-2   hard

536 Broadway, New York, NY 10012-3955 • (212) 431-4370
Fax (212) 941-7842 • Order Toll-Free: (877) 687-7476 • www.springerpub.com

BREAST CANCER
Journey to Recovery

Carol Noll Hoskins, PhD, RN, FAAN
Judith Haber, PhD, APRN, CS, FAAN
Wendy Budin, PhD, RN, C

This book portrays the personal experience of breast cancer through the stories of three women and their partners. The combination of emotional and factual information on the disease, treatment options, and health promotion, makes this important reading for health professionals and their patients. It is derived from a major NYU Nursing study of 121 couples. Each chapter is followed by study questions and a knowledge review, which can be used in patient education. An overview of the NYU study is given as well as a list of relevant internet sites. (A companion video series is also available.)

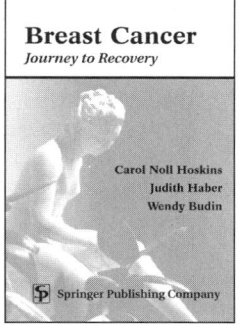

Contents:
• Preface
• **Chapter I:** Coping With A Diagnosis of Breast Cancer
• **Chapter II:** Recovering From Surgery
• **Chapter III:** Understanding Adjuvant Therapy
• **Chapter IV:** Ongoing Recovery
• **Chapter V:** A Program of Research: Education, Counseling, and Adjustment Among Breast Cancer Patients and Partners
• Appendix: Information Resources

2001   128pp   0-8261-1392-3   soft

SPRINGER PUBLISHING COMPANY • www.springerpub.com
Order Toll-Free: 877.687.7476 • Phone: 212.431.4370 • Fax: 212.941.7842